THE
VINEGAR
BIBLE

How This Ancient Elixir
Cleanses Your Body & Slashes Fat

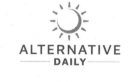

ALTERNATIVE
DAILY

CONTENTS

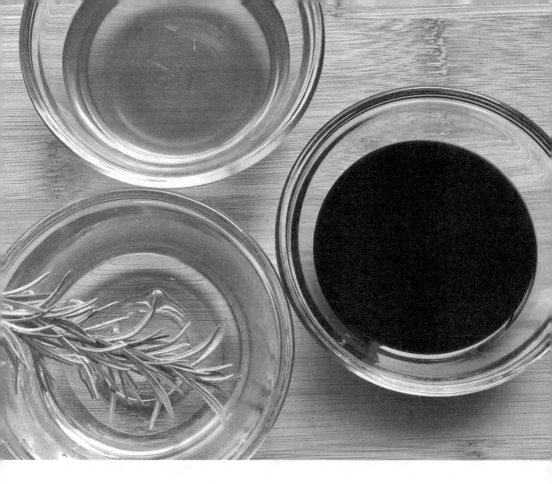

Introduction

Vinegar is one of the most essential items anyone can have in their kitchen pantry. Not only is it one of the most versatile ingredients to use in a wide variety of dishes, but without it, your favorite salad dressings and many other foods just wouldn't be the same. And, your pickles? Well, they wouldn't be pickled now, would they?

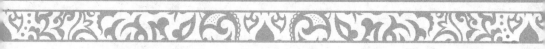

Vinegar offers a multitude of health benefits too. And when it comes to adding flavor without sugar, fat or a lot of calories, it truly is your best friend. The word "vinegar" comes from the French word *vin egre*, which means "sour wine." It's been produced and sold for thousands of years, dating back to some time before the 6th century BCE. Hippocrates was said to have used it to help heal wounds quicker, while Babylonians were known to use vinegars flavored with fruit, honey and malt. The ancient Chinese even used it to prevent infection and clean their hands.

Throughout history, vinegar has proven to be the most versatile of products. The dictionary defines versatile as "capable of turning with ease from one thing to another," and for the past 10,000 years or so, humans have used it in several different ways. Through the centuries vinegar has been produced from many other materials including molasses, dates, sorghum, fruits, berries, melons, coconut, honey, beer, maple syrup, potatoes, beets, malt, grains and whey, but the primary part of the process remains unchanged: fermentation.

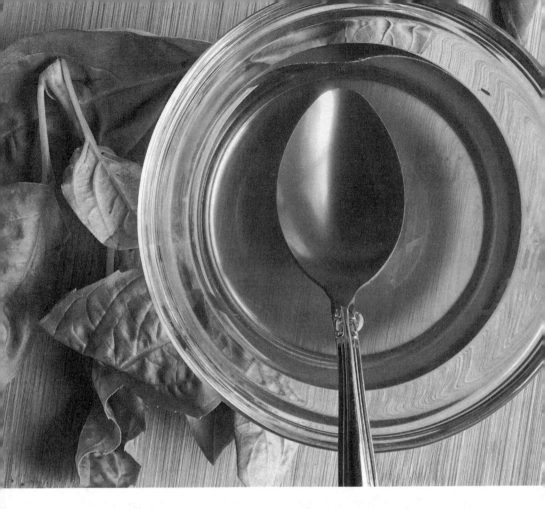

Vinegar is made by bacterial activity that transforms fermented liquids like cider and wine into a weak solution of acetic acid — that acetic acid is what gives vinegar its pungent smell. Any ingredient containing ethanol can be used to make vinegar, including cider, wine distilled grain alcohol, champagne, beer and more. The acetic acid makes vinegar unique, although it contains other substances including vitamins, minerals and flavor compounds. The bacterial culture used to ferment the ethanol is referred to as the "mother of vinegar."

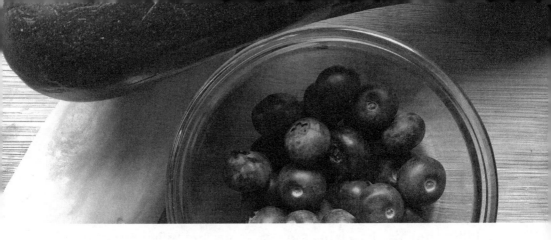

Pasteurized vinegar has been heat-treated to kill the "mother" culture, which can form a slime-like glob of cellulose that has a cobweb-like appearance in the vinegar. Most types of vinegar meant for consumption have been pasteurized to prevent this slime from occurring, as consumers are often put off by it. Stopping the bacteria via pasteurization also helps maintain product consistency. Varieties of vinegar that have not been pasteurized are often labeled as "raw." Today, thanks to much scientific research over the years, we know that vinegar is rich in bioactive compounds. It not only contains acetic acid, but gallic acid, catechin, epicatechin, caffeic acid and more, which is what gives it such powerful antioxidant and antimicrobial properties, along with many other benefits.

Vinegar remains popular around the world today for pickling fruits and vegetables, and it's also commonly added to condiments and other food dishes for flavor. It's also become increasingly popular as a health tonic, particularly unpasteurized vinegar that still contains the "mother."

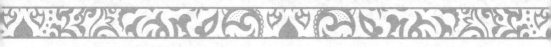

Vinegars are purported to treat numerous diseases, illnesses and other health issues, such as preventing premature aging, relieving digestive woes, healing acne, lowering inflammation, killing fungus, dissolving kidney stones and relieving numerous other ailments like allergies, heartburn, migraines and asthma, as well as aiding the body in detoxification.

It's intriguing to think that in today's modern, high-tech world, we're still using one product that was discovered over 10,000 years ago when, reportedly, someone found a cask of wine that had gone past its time and had been transformed into this wonderful new food.

The United States Food and Drug Administration (FDA) requires that any product called "vinegar" contain at least four percent acidity. This ensures the minimum strength of the vinegar sold at retailers. There are currently no standards of identity for vinegar, but the FDA has established "Compliance Policy Guides" that it follows regarding labeling of vinegars like cider, wine, malt, sugar, spirit and vinegar blends. In other places, like Europe, each has their own regional standards for vinegar produced or sold in the area.

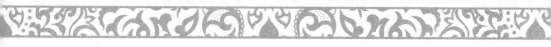

Ancient Use

With such a long, rich history, vinegar has been used by many ancient populations, from the Sumerians of Babylonia to modern humans around the globe today. Vinegar residues have even been discovered in urns from ancient Egypt and were traced back to 3,000 BCE.

The timeline that begins with its discovery is arguably the best way to understand its fascinating history. Vinegar, which was believed to be discovered more than 10,000 years ago, has evolved tremendously throughout the times due to its impressive uses.

Ancient Babylonia

While there are no records of vinegar before 5,000 BCE, legend has it that the Sumerians, a civilization of Ancient Babylonia, used vinegar for cleaning on a day-to-day basis throughout their lives. Because they found that it could stop or slow the action of bacteria that spoils food, they began using it as a preservative, as well as a condiment.

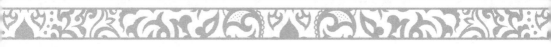

Ancient Egypt

Some 2,000 years later, the Egyptians were using vinegar too — something that was revealed when archaeologists found the urns dating back to 3,000 BCE which still contained remnants of it. Queen Cleopatra, born in 69 BCE, who went on to become one of history's most famous rulers, was said to have showed off the solvency powers of vinegar by dissolving precious pearls in the liquid to win a bet with Marc Antony where she said she'd consume the fortune, literally, in a single meal.

Although there are many tomb drawings and small models that represent agriculture, kitchen activities and banquets during this period, knowledge of specific ways by which food was prepared is practically non-existent. However, there are a few clues that are contained in the hieratic inscriptions found on various shards of pottery, known as ostrica. Through millennia, ostrica were used like paper in order to record all types of information, which, today, provides a glimpse into the daily life of the times. A receipt discovered for various services rendered, written during the reign of Ramses II (1279–1213 BCE), records payment for services — and all were made in jars of what's believed to be vinegar.

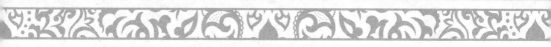

Ancient China

The first confirmed written history of vinegar in China dates to 1200 BCE. By 479 BCE, large scale vinegar manufacturing is believed to have already begun. In the city of Jinyang, modern day Taiyuan, there were reportedly several different vinegar manufacturers in the city, according to Chinese historian Hao Shuhou. By then, vinegar had grown to become more than just a casually made condiment, as evidenced by the fact that the royal courts of many Chinese states had a special position for a person with the sole responsibility of brewing vinegar for royal consumption.

In the early 1970s, a medical text dating back to the Qin/Han Dynasties of the 3rd century BCE was discovered by Chinese archaeologists. Known as "Recipes for the 52 Ailments," it describes treatments for many common conditions from snakebites to ulcers to venereal disease. While many of the ingredients are herbal and are still mainstays of Chinese medicine, they often included vinegar as the main or accompanying ingredient.

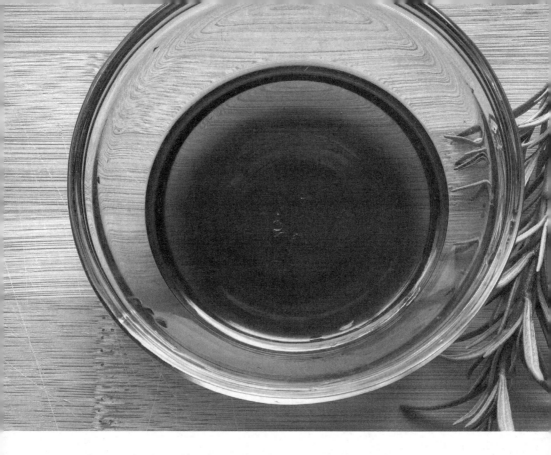

Ancient Greece

The use of vinegar to fight infections and other acute conditions dates back to Hippocrates, 460 to 377 BCE. The father of medicine was said to have recommended a vinegar preparation for cleaning ulcerations as well as to treat sores. A popular ancient medicine known as oxymel, made up of honey and vinegar, was prescribed for persistent coughs by Hippocrates and his contemporaries, and by physicians up to modern day.

Ancient Rome

The Romans used to drink "posca," a mix of water and vinegar that was sold in the streets, similarly to coconut sellers today. It was believed to give strength. A sponge soaked in posca was even said to have been offered by a praetorian to Jesus on the cross as a sign of mercy. In Roman banquets, a bowl containing a glass and a half of vinegar, known as acetabulum, was used by diners to soak small pieces of bread during a meal to improve digestion. Nearly all recipes created by famous Epicurean gastronomist Apicius contained vinegar, and the Romans have used several types of vinegar in sauces as well as for dressing vegetables and salads.

The Romans were the ones who introduced the marinating process to keep fried fish, while Plinius the Elder recommended vinegar in his "Naturalis Historia" to treat a number of conditions and improve life in general. Julius Caesar, one of the most famous of all Roman generals, made his armies drink vinegar as a beverage. It was also used by the Carthaginian general Hannibal when he crossed the Alps with elephants to invade Italy in 218 BCE, by pouring it hot over boulders to crumble them, which allowed his troops to march through.

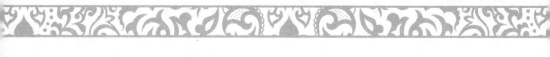

The Middle Ages

During the Middle Ages, from the 5th to the 15th century, vinegar was used in many different, often extraordinary ways. During the Black Plague, from the mid-14th century to the late 18th century, physicians rubbed vinegar infused with herbs and essential oils across their bodies to protect themselves from germs while attending to those who were contagious. Thieves used it the same way, often drinking large amounts infused with garlic in order to avoid catching the disease before robbing the dead. In the 17th century, many Europeans used vinegar as a deodorizer. They would soak sponges in it and then hold it up to their noses to reduce the smell of raw sewage in the street. The sponges were carried by the men in their walking canes, and by the women in tiny silver boxes.

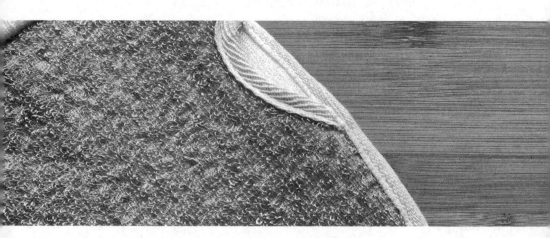

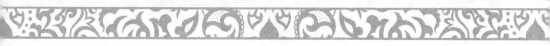

It was also in the Middle Ages that vinegar started being used, along with an abrasive material like sand, to clean and polish flexible mail armor. In 1394, a group of French winemakers developed a continuous method for making vinegar, known as the Orleans method. In this method, oak barrels were used as fermentation vessels and the vinegar was siphoned off through a spigot at the bottom of the barrel. About 15 percent of the vinegar was left behind, which contained the "mother" of vinegar and its concentrated bacteria floating on top. A new batch of cider or wine was then carefully added to the barrel, which was quick-started by the remaining vinegar. These early French vintners formed a guild of master vinegar makers, and by utilizing the Orleans method, they were better able to supply the profitable vinegar market.

19th and 20th Centuries

Throughout history, the antiseptic nature of vinegar has been used to clean and disinfect the wounds of soldiers to speed up wound healing. It was used this way during the American Civil War and as late as the First World War.

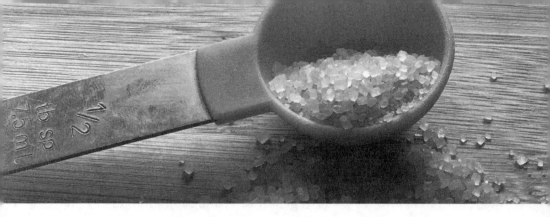

13 Well-Known And Less Common Vinegars (And How To Make Some)

While you're probably very familiar with vinegars like apple cider vinegar, white distilled, red wine vinegar and balsamic vinegar, you may be surprised to learn that there are actually dozens of different types of vinegars.

While the most common, apple cider and white distilled, are considered pantry staples, the more adventurous might want to try some of the lesser known vinegars like rice vinegar, Champagne vinegar and gourmet varieties, such as a rich black fig vinegar. These days, you can find vinegars infused with all types of flavors, from mango and peach to dark chocolate and even espresso. Vinegars can be made from just about any food that contains natural sugars. Yeast ferments these sugars into alcohol, and certain types of bacteria convert that alcohol a second time into vinegar. A weak acetic acid remains after the

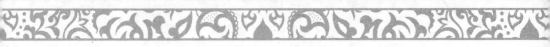

second fermentation. The acid contains flavors reminiscent of the original fermented food, like apples or grapes. Acetic acid is what gives vinegar its distinct aroma and taste.

On a basic level, vinegar is acetic acid produced by the fermentation of an alcoholic liquid by acetic acid bacteria. Nearly every region in the world, including China, India, Italy, Austria, France and well beyond, has fermented some ingredient, like dates, coconut, rice, persimmon, honey and beer, to create a vinegar. Vinegars are virtually calorie free. Those that have some added sugar, like malt and balsamic, may have a small amount, but still hardly anything worth counting, which means sugar and fat are virtually nonexistent too. Only vinegars with added salt, such as seasoned rice vinegar, have any sodium. It's one of those rare food items in the world that we can actually consider a "freebie," and as such, why not take advantage of its many uses?

Of course, with so many different types of vinegars, and such an overwhelming amount of uses, it can be hard to know where to begin. We'll make it a little easier on you by providing this "guided tour" to the world of common vinegars — and some of the less common too.

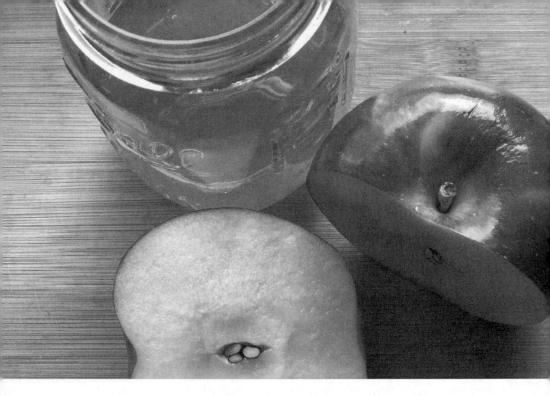

Common Vinegars

. . . .

Apple Cider Vinegar

Apple Cider Vinegar, or ACV, is the vinegar that's most widely hailed for its nutritive properties, both for consumption and topical use, particularly, the unpasteurized, raw organic apple cider vinegar that still contains the "mother." This means ACV that still has the culture of beneficial bacteria which turns regular apple cider into vinegar in the first place, similar to the SCOBY (also referred to as the mother) in making kombucha.

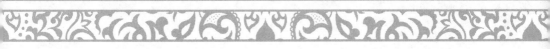

The mother is a complex structure of beneficial acids that provide a host of health benefits. Most unrefined vinegars have a murky appearance due to this mother culture. Clear and pasteurized vinegars typically do not contain the mother culture and don't carry the same benefits.

This type of ACV is purported to treat numerous diseases, illnesses and other health issues. Among its very long list of abilities, it's said to promote healthier cholesterol levels, reduce excess inflammation, kill fungus, prevent premature aging, dissolve kidney stones, relieve heartburn as well as migraines, asthma and allergy symptoms. It can also be used topically to treat acne, nail fungus and bug bites as well as to promote younger looking skin. It gives the skin a healthy glow, promoting improved circulation which brings more oxygen and nutrients to the skin's surface.

Of course, apple cider vinegar has many culinary uses too. It adds a tarty, tangy flavor to things like marinades and salad dressings as well as seasoning vegetables, and is considered an all-purpose pantry staple. As ACV is one of the most common and beneficial of all vinegars, you may even want to consider

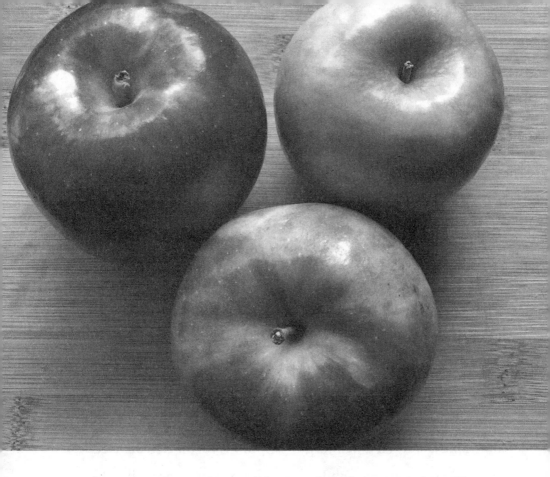

making your own at home. It's surprisingly easy and you'll save a lot of cash too. This is a job that's best done in the fall, which will allow you to take advantage of the seasonal bounty of apples. While visiting an apple orchard can be a lot of fun, if you don't have one near you, you can always pick up a bag of organic apples from your local co-op, a farmers market or grocery store.

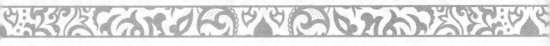

Types of apples to use for making ACV

A mixture of various types of apples generally produces the best tasting and most healthful raw apple cider vinegar. To start out, you might want to use these approximate ratios, and then you can change it up as desired to suit personal preferences for later batches:

- 50 percent sweet apples, like Fuji, golden delicious, red delicious and gala

- 35 percent sharp tasting apples, such as Granny Smith and McIntosh

- 15 percent bitter tasting apples, like Cortland, Newtown and Dolgo crabapples

In some places, more bitter apples can be challenging to find. If it's the case where you are, you can increase the proportion of sweet apples to 60 percent and the sharp tasting apples to 40 percent. While the flavor won't be as complex, it will still be beneficial healthwise and have a good taste as well.

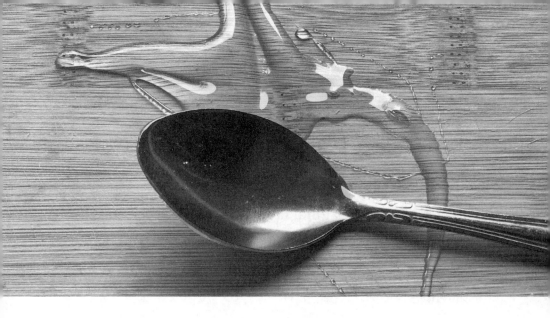

Here's what you'll need to make it:

- ☑ 5 large apples of choice, or the scraps of 10 apples, with a ratio as described above
- ☑ Filtered water
- ☑ 1 cup raw, local honey
- ☑ 1 wide mouth gallon glass jar
- ☑ Cheesecloth
- ☑ A large rubber band

Before you can make your raw apple cider vinegar, you'll first need to make hard apple cider. The alcohol in the hard cider is what transforms via fermentation into acetic acid, which is the beneficial organic compound that gives apple cider vinegar its sour taste.

1. Wash your apples and coarsely chop them into pieces no smaller than an inch. You can include the seeds, stems and cores if you'd like.

2. Place your chopped apples into the gallon glass jar. Never brew the vinegar in stainless steel pots, as the vinegar will cause leaching of heavy metals (like carcinogenic nickel) to the acidity. Be sure your apples fill half the jar, and perhaps a bit more. If it's not halfway full after you've added the chopped apples, you can add apple scraps until it is.

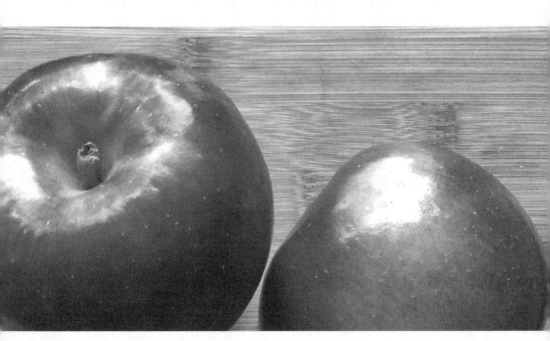

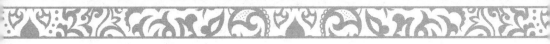

3. Pour in filtered water (room temperature) until the apples are totally covered and the jar is nearly full. A couple of inches should be left at the top.

4. Stir in raw honey until it has completely dissolved.

5. Cover the top of the jar with cheesecloth and then secure it with a large rubber band.

6. Leave the jar on your kitchen counter for one to two weeks, mixing it gently once or twice each day throughout this period. Bubbles will start to form when the sugar ferments into alcohol — you'll be able to smell this process.

7. When the apple scraps are no longer floating and sink to the bottom of the jar (usually between one and two weeks at most), your hard apple cider is ready. If they still haven't sunk after two weeks, but the mixture has the smell of alcohol, it's okay to move onto the next step.

8. Strain out the apple scraps and then pour the hard apple cider into a clean, one gallon glass jar or into smaller sized mason jars. Cover with a fresh piece of cheesecloth and secure the jar (or jars) with a rubberband.

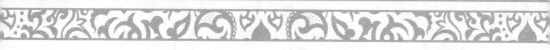

9. Leave the jar on your kitchen counter for an additional three to four weeks. This allows the alcohol to be converted into acetic acid, thanks to the action of healthy bacteria. A small amount of sediment on the bottom is normal. The mother culture should form on top.

10. After three weeks, taste the raw apple cider vinegar to determine if it's ready. If it has the desired taste, you can strain it one more time and then store it inside clean, glass mason jars or jugs. If after four weeks the taste still isn't quite strong enough, leave it for another week and then taste it again. If you accidentally leave it too long and the taste is too strong, you can still use it. Simply strain and dilute it with some water to a level of acidity that you prefer.

Store your apple cider vinegar in a pantry or cabinet out of direct sunlight. While it won't go bad, if you do leave it for a long time, another mother culture will likely form on the top. If the taste is too strong, you can simply strain it again and dilute it using a little water.

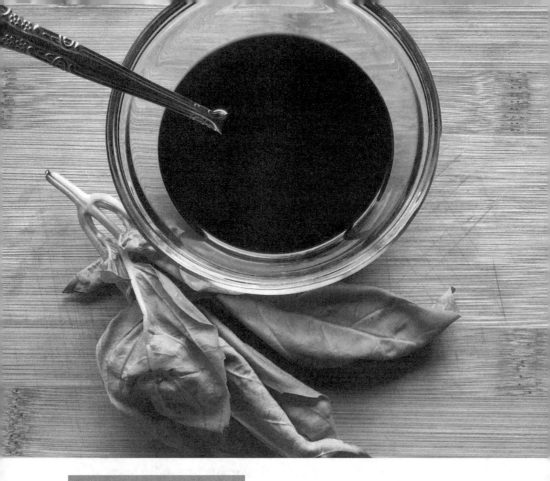

Balsamic Vinegar

Balsamic vinegar is known around the world to cooks and is widely available in grocery stores. It can be as inexpensive as a few dollars for a 16-ounce bottle or as much as $200 an ounce because of the wide differences between varieties. We'll discuss traditional balsamic vinegar, the most common of balsamic vinegars. It's made only in Modena and Reggio Emilia, Italy, using traditional methods. All production is overseen from start to finish by a special certification agency.

This vinegar starts with grape must, whole pressed, late-harvested white grapes that include the skin, seeds, stems and juice. It's cooked over a direct flame until concentrated, by roughly half. Then, it's allowed to naturally ferment for up to three weeks before being matured and further concentrated for at least 12 years in five or more successively smaller aging

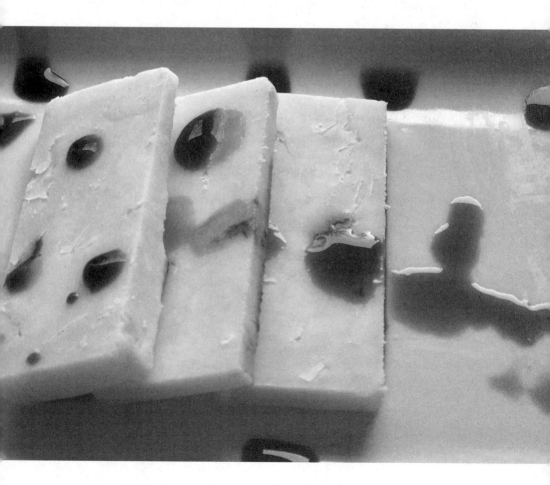

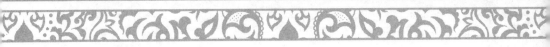

barrels. The barrels are made from various types of wood, like chestnut, mulberry, juniper and oak, which results in the vinegar taking on the complex flavors of the casks. The vinegar gets thicker and more concentrated as it ages because of evaporation that occurs through the walls of the barrels.

Traditional balsamic vinegar has a rich, complex sweetness, with notes of cherry, fig, prune, molasses or even chocolate. It has a mellow tartness instead of strong acidity, and moves a bit like syrup with a velvety texture. It's not used as a cooking ingredient, as heating kills its distinctive bouquet. Using it as an ingredient in a dressing is not recommended generally either, as it's flavors would be wasted. Instead, drizzle it on salty foods like goat cheese, or onto fruits like fresh strawberries or raspberries. You can even add a few drops onto vanilla ice cream or another type of creamy dessert.

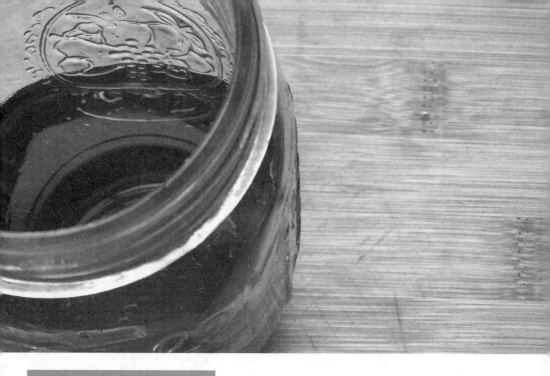

Red Wine Vinegar

Red wine vinegar is an excellent all-purpose vinegar that's considered a pantry staple for use in marinades, salad dressings and more. It's the result of the more traditional vinegar making process, utilizing wine for the bacteria to ferment. It offers an obvious visual contribution, which is why it's most commonly used in heartier dishes such as a marinade for red meat or in barbecue and marinara sauces. A good red wine vinegar can be hard to find; the type in grocery stores is often too acidic. In addition, specialty food shops carry more fancy balsamic and flavored vinegars, but rarely top-shelf red wine varieties. So, this is another vinegar you may want to make on your own.

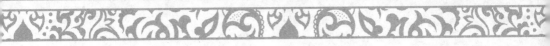

To make red wine vinegar, you'll need:

- ☑ A piece of the "mother," sold at wine and beer-making supply stores
- ☑ 750-ml bottle of red wine to start, small amount more needed weekly for 3 months
- ☑ 2 cups water
- ☑ Cheesecloth

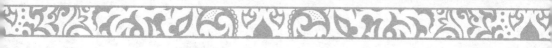

Here's how to do it:

Place the piece of the mother into a wide-mouth, gallon glass container. Add the contents of the bottle of red wine and the two cups of water. Secure a double-layered piece of cheesecloth over the top and then place it into a cool, dark spot.

1. Every week, add a little more red wine, gently pushing the mother aside each time.

2. After about three months, taste the mixture. If it tastes like vinegar, strain it into clean containers and allow it to age for anywhere from one to six months. In order to keep the liquid clear and prevent a new mother from forming, you can pasteurize it by pouring it into a pot and diluting it with water according to preference. Heat it until it reaches 155°F by using an instant-read thermometer. Maintain that temperature for 30 minutes.

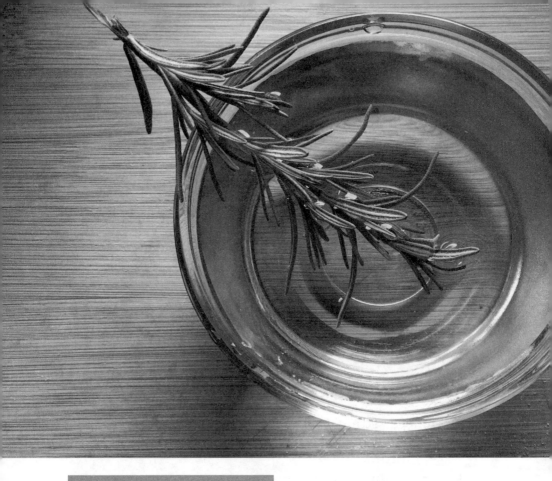

White Wine Vinegar

White wine vinegar is different from harsh distilled white vinegar. While it isn't as flavorful as its red counterpart, it lightens and brightens rich sauces and vinaigrettes without overpowering the other flavors in the dish. Made from white wine, the taste is more mellow. It is often used for fish and poultry, as well as recipes where you don't want to change the color.

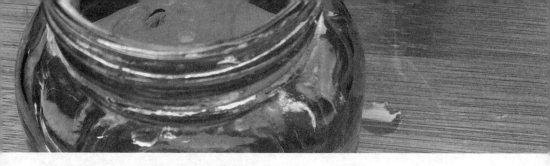

White Distilled Vinegar

This vinegar is generally the cheapest and most widely available. It's typically made from malt or corn and fermented to produce the vinegar. It's distinctly different from white wine vine vinegar and the most commonly used in commercial production for things like bottled salad dressings, pickles and ketchup. Because of its high level of acidity, it's more frequently utilized for things other than consumption, such as household cleaning, drain cleaner, disinfectants, pesticides and as an Easter egg dye medium.

Malt Vinegar

Malt vinegar is fermented from malted barley. It's brewed from beer and then allowed to ferment and age briefly. Malt vinegar is most commonly associated with fish and chips as a popular condiment, especially in the United Kingdom. It's also good for pickling, chutneys and other recipes like salt and vinegar potatoes or glazed chicken. Caution: For people who need to be gluten-free, malt vinegar is not a good choice because it is not gluten-free.

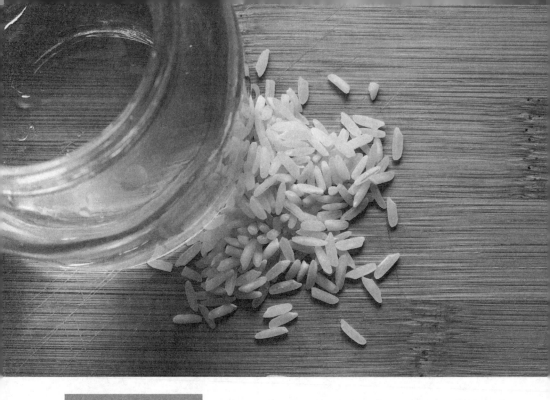

Rice Vinegar

Rice vinegar is considered a staple in Southeast Asian cooking, thanks to its low acetic acid content, which adds a light flavor ideal for drizzling on vegetables like tomatoes or cucumbers, in stir-fries and on salads. It's most commonly produced in Japan and China from rice wine that's allowed to ferment. It has a sweeter taste than wine vinegars, while being less harsh than white distilled vinegar.

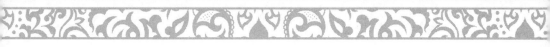

Sherry Vinegar

Sherry vinegar is made from sherry wine, a fortified wine that's left to mature for at least six months (and sometimes for years) in oak barrels before being bottled. Made in Spain, it's known for having one of the most deep, complex flavors of all wine vinegars. It's great to use as a vinaigrette as well as flavoring stews and sauces.

Champagne Vinegar

Champagne vinegar is often combined with fruit vinegars to create a variety of vinaigrettes. It is excellent for sauces, dressings and marinades. Made from Champagne, France, it has a fresher, lighter taste as compared to other wine vinegars. It's easy to make too! If you happen to have leftover Champagne (which quickly loses its fizzle), you can use it to make vinegar instead of tossing it out.

To make Champagne vinegar, pour Champagne into wide-mouthed jars and leave them open. After three weeks, the resulting vinegar can be used to make vinaigrette. It can then be stored and covered for up to six months.

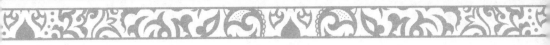

Lesser Known Types of Vinegar

There are a number of more unique, less common vinegars you might want to experiment with, too.

Coconut Vinegar

Both coconuts and vinegar are highly popular today for their medicinal benefits. Fortunately, you can take advantage of both of them in coconut vinegar. It's most often used in Thai cooking for marinades and sauces, and has a slightly yeasty, strong, sharp taste.

The key to utilizing the maximum potential of coconut vinegar's benefits is to choose those that are based in coconut sap, as coconut water isn't as concentrated and doesn't contain nearly as many enzymes and natural probiotics. Coconut sap vinegar contains all nine essential amino acids and eight non-essential amino acids, which offer numerous health benefits, such as helping to fight infection and support the immune system. It's also packed with some 65 different minerals.

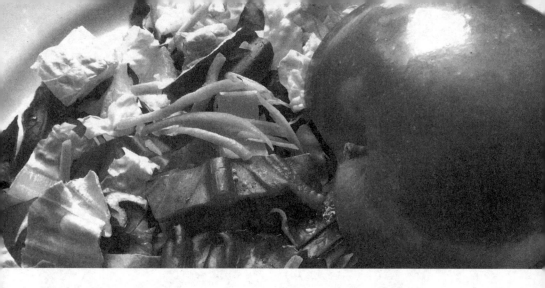

Use coconut vinegar like you would apple cider vinegar; the options are practically endless. It's less pungent than ACV, but still has the flavor of vinegar. You can add it as an ingredient in a homemade salad dressing, or use it in sauces and marinades. It can also be used as a health tonic by mixing a tablespoon of coconut vinegar with a tablespoon of water and drinking it in the morning when you wake up, on an empty stomach. It's said to help improve digestion and boost energy throughout the day.

Coconut vinegar can also be made with ingredients that you probably already have in your kitchen, though it's best done by fermenting coconut water with yeast and sugar. All you have to do is strain the coconut water through cheesecloth, add the sugar and stir well. Boil the mixture to 149°F for 20 minutes, and then place it into a clean mason jar. Add the yeast and then set it aside for one week. It's ready when it smells acidic and is slightly foamy.

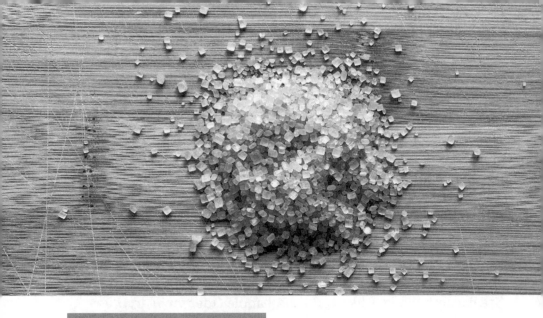

Sugar Cane Vinegar

Sugar Cane Vinegar is slightly sweet and acidic. It's a staple in Indian kitchens, widely used in chutneys and for pickling. This vinegar is made from the syrup of sugar cane, which is harvested and crushed to extract the juice and then simmered down into a syrup. The syrup is then fermented into vinegar — the best sugar cane vinegars are also aged in oak barrels. It has a more mellow flavor, like malt vinegar. It's not sweet and it is much less harsh than distilled vinegars.

Spirit Vinegar

The strongest of all vinegars, this is used almost exclusively for pickling. It differs from distilled vinegar in that it contains a small quantity of alcohol.

Flavored Vinegars

Flavored vinegars have been around for centuries. All types of things have been added to vinegar to infuse it with flavor, from herbs and spices to fruits, berries and beyond. The options are practically endless, and really only limited to one's imagination. They include unique vinegars like espresso vinegar, which takes advantage of many a chef's "secret ingredient," coffee, to bring its rich, sweet complex flavors to dishes like steaks, chops and chicken or to add richness to grilled meats. There are mango and peach vinegars that are wonderful to drizzle on greens. There are even dark chocolate vinegars, ideal on red meats.

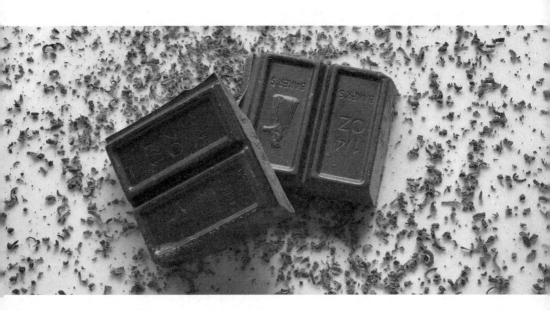

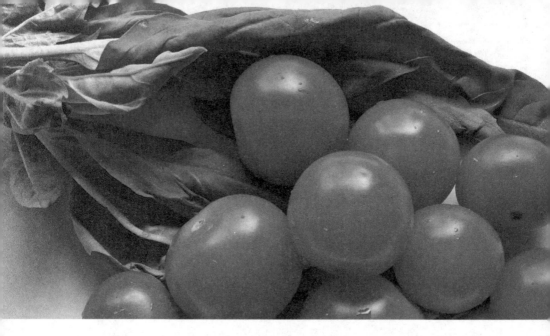

Vinegar and Your Health

As mentioned earlier, the health benefits of vinegar are nothing new. As early as 400 BCE, Hippocrates, the famous ancient Greek physician, used fruit-derived vinegars to remedy wounds, coughs and more.

Today, vinegar still remains in the spotlight regarding its therapeutic capabilities. While we hear a lot about apple cider vinegar, other grain and fruit vinegars are being studied for their beneficial physiological effects that include antibacterial and antioxidant properties. A 2016 review in the journal of *Comprehensive Reviews in Food Science and Food Safety* notes that some vinegars (particularly Japanese black soybean vinegar) even have anticancer properties.

Here are just some of the ways vinegar may improve your health.

Blood sugar regulation

A 2015 study in the *Journal of Diabetes Research* found that when people with type 2 diabetes consumed one ounce of vinegar mixed with 20 milliliters of water before a meal, their blood glucose, insulin and triglyceride levels were lower for up to five hours after a meal compared to a placebo. In addition, those who consumed the vinegar had a greater uptake of insulin from the blood which is also helpful for blood sugar regulation.

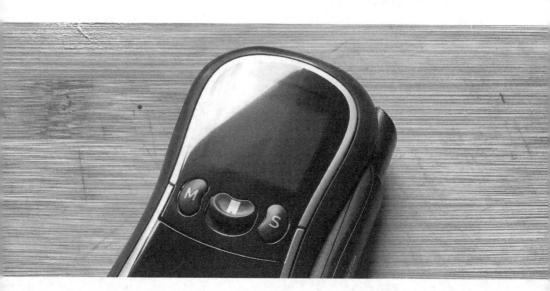

Another study, published in the *European Journal of Clinical Nutrition*, found that people who had impaired glucose had improved blood flow in their muscles, improved glucose uptake by muscles and reduced blood insulin and triglyceride levels up to five hours after the meal. Researchers noted that, "Vinegar may be considered beneficial for improving insulin resistance and metabolic abnormalities in people with prediabetes."

Heart health

Balsamic vinegar prevents low-density lipoproteins (LDL) from oxidizing, which is thought to contribute to the buildup of plaque on artery walls.

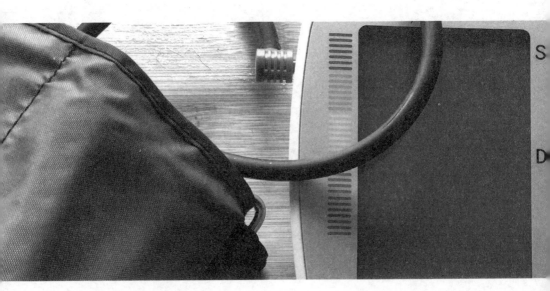

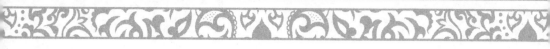

Bacteria fighter

The antibacterial properties of vinegar can help fight infection causing a sore throat. Vinegar's acidity helps decrease the tissue pH and prevents bacteria from growing. A 2014 study found that the acetic acid found in vinegar also acts as a non-toxic disinfectant against drug-resistant tuberculosis bacteria.

Clean an infection with vinegar

This old-time method of cleaning out wounds is effective and even fun for kids. Sprinkle baking soda over the area and pour a little vinegar over it. Soak the infected part in warm water for 15 minutes.

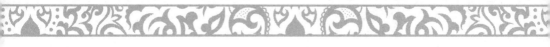

Cider Cough Drops

These cough drops can help ease the pain of a sore throat and reduce coughing.

- ☑ 2 tbsp organic butter
- ☑ 1/2 cup seasoned rice vinegar
- ☑ 2 cups sugar

1. Melt the butter in a medium-size saucepan (on medium heat) and add sugar and vinegar.

2. Stir constantly. Tip: Brush down the inside of the pot with a pastry brush dipped in cold water. This will keep the mixture from sticking to the sides of the pan.

3. Boil the mixture on high for up to ten minutes. As it thickens it will turn white colored.

4. Remove mixture from the heat and spread on pieces of oiled aluminum foil. Once it cools and become brittle, break it apart into small pieces.

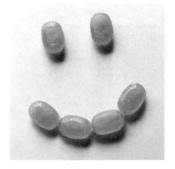

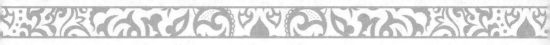

Vinegar Cough Syrup

Take two tablespoons of this cough remedy at first sign of a cough and at bedtime.

- ☑ 1/2 cup cider vinegar
- ☑ 1/2 cup filtered water
- ☑ 1 tsp cayenne pepper
- ☑ 1/4 cup honey

Weight loss

Using vinegar as a substitute for many higher calorie condiments, such as salad dressing, can help you maintain or even lose weight.

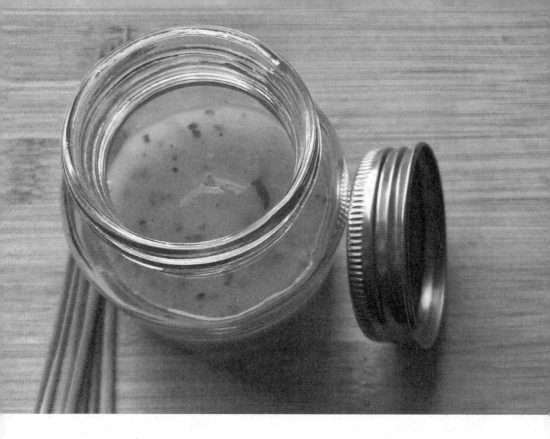

Simple Vinegar Salad Dressing

- ☑ 1 part vinegar of your choice
- ☑ 3 parts oil
- ☑ 1 tbsp raw honey
- ☑ Juice of 1 lemon
- ☑ Fresh chopped herbs of your choice

Add all ingredients in a glass jar and shake well before using. Store in the fridge for up to one week.

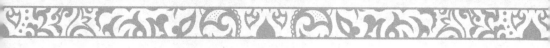

Raw Apple Cider Vinaigrette

- ☑ 1/2 cup apple cider vinegar
- ☑ 1/2 cup grapeseed oil
- ☑ 2 tbsp of pure maple syrup
- ☑ Salt and pepper to taste

Mix all ingredients in a mason jar and shake gently. Store in the refrigerator for up to a week.

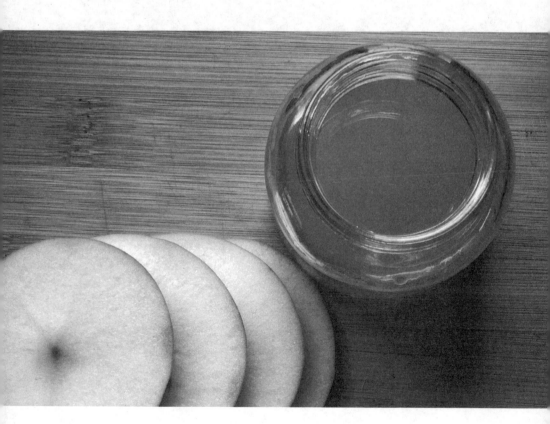

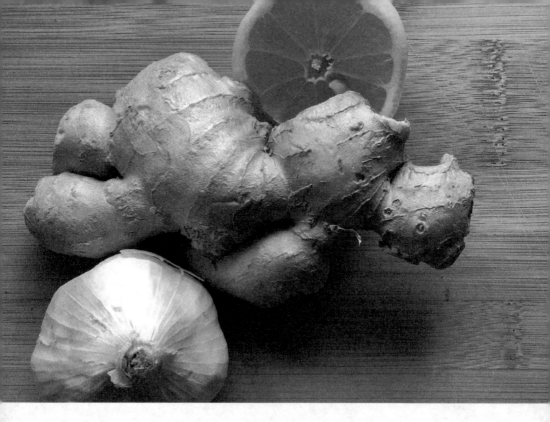

Garlic and Ginger Dressing

- ☑ 1/2 cup apple cider vinegar
- ☑ 1/4 cup extra virgin olive oil
- ☑ 1/4 cup sesame oil
- ☑ 2 tbsp fresh grated ginger
- ☑ 1 tbsp fresh lemon
- ☑ I tsp minced garlic

Mix all ingredients together in a glass jar and shake lightly.
Store in refrigerator for up to a week.

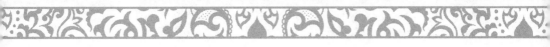

Nutrient absorption

Including apple cider vinegar in meals or drinking a mild tonic of vinegar and water (one tablespoon of vinegar in a glass of water) just before or with your meal can help your body absorb important minerals locked in foods. This is especially helpful for women who have a hard time getting enough calcium.

Calcium Supplement

Rather than taking a conventional supplement, try making your own.

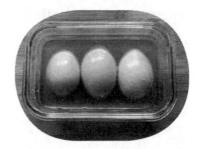

- ☑ 4 raw eggs
- ☑ Cider vinegar

1. Wash the eggs and put them in a glass bowl.

2. Cover them with cider vinegar and let them set for two days until the shell is dissolved. Remove the raw eggs for another use.

3. Stir the remaining liquid and store in a small glass jar with a lid. Take one tablespoon each day with a glass of water.

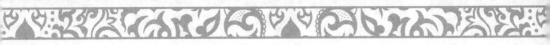

Cancer

As mentioned, vinegar may help reduce the risk of cancer. This is due to the fact that vinegars are a very rich source of polyphenols, plant compounds that fight oxidative stress.

Brain health

Could vinegar make you smarter? Some say that consuming vinegar may help with cognitive function. Research shows that acetic acid bacteria produce precursors of very important building blocks of brain tissues known as sphingolipids.

Injuries

The "mother" of vinegar, which is found in unprocessed, unfiltered vinegar, is loaded with antibacterial properties that can help speed healing of burns. In addition, consuming acetic acid bacteria may also help minimize muscle damage from inflammation after exercise.

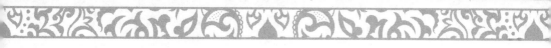

More Home Remedies Using Vinegar

Here are some additional ways that you can use vinegar for health and wellbeing.

Cold Fixer

Mix 1/4 cup apple cider vinegar and 1/4 cup raw honey together in eight ounces of warm water. Take this mixture by the tablespoon six times a day.

Mucus Buster

To cut mucus, mix equal parts raw honey with vinegar and take one tablespoon at a time.

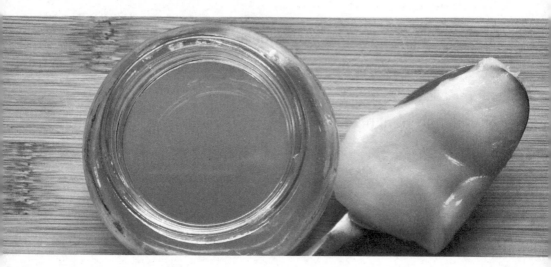

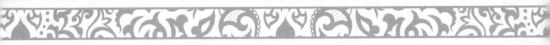

Breathe Easy

Add 1/4 cup vinegar to vaporizer water to help open air passages.

Digestive Aid

Make your own peppermint vinegar by placing a few peppermint leaves in a small jar of cider vinegar and letting it infuse for a few days. Strain the mixture into a clean glass jar and add three teaspoons of honey. Stir a few spoonfuls of the peppermint vinegar in a glass of warm water and drink to ease an upset stomach.

Athlete's Foot Healer

Soak your feet in equal parts vinegar and warm water to eliminate athlete's foot. You can also add a few drops of tea tree essential oil to the water. You can also spray your feet with full strength vinegar a few times a day.

Warts Be Gone

Apply a solution of equal parts cider vinegar and glycerin to warts daily until they are gone.

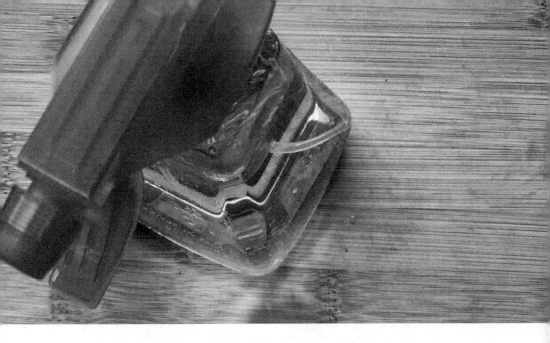

Jelly Fish Sting Reliever

Reduce the pain, sting, itch and inflammation of a jelly fish
bite by spraying full strength white vinegar on the impacted
area.

Insect Bite Paste

To treat insect bites, make a paste with cornstarch and
vinegar and apply to the affected area.

Sunburn Soother

Cover sunburn in a light cotton towel soaked in vinegar. This
will help reduce inflammation and cool your skin. You can
also add a few ice cubes to a spray bottle full of vinegar and
spray on sunburned areas to ease pain.

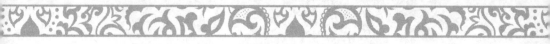

Yeast Infection Remedy

Add two cups of vinegar to bath water to remedy yeast infections in girls and women.

Hemorrhoid Helper

Soak cotton balls in vinegar, then dab directly on hemorrhoids to ease pain and swelling.

Wind Protector

If you are going to be out in the wind, apply a very light layer of olive oil thinned with vinegar on your face. This will serve as a protective barrier against the elements.

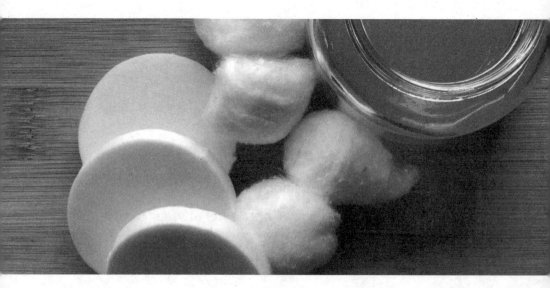

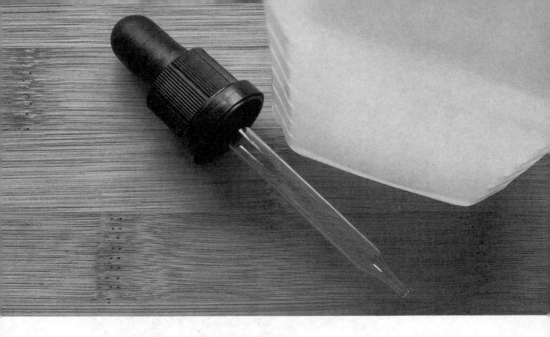

Swimmer's Ear Treatment

If you are prone to swimmer's ear, you can kill bacteria and fungus that lurks in the outer ear canal. Mix together equal parts of vinegar and alcohol, then put two drops in each ear after swimming. Allow the liquid to drain after one minute.

Note: When using vinegar for health it is important not to use distilled white vinegar. While this type of vinegar is great for cleaning, it offers very little for health. Always choose organic, unfiltered and unprocessed vinegar for health applications. This vinegar is not sparkling clean but rather murky and includes a cobweb-like substance known as "mother."

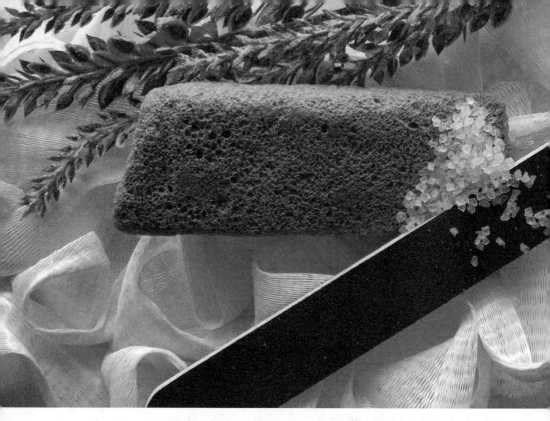

Grooming and Beauty

Just as vinegar can be an effective remedy for a number of troubling conditions, it can also be an amazing addition to your grooming and beauty regime.

To condition your hair, add natural highlights and keep dandruff away, make a rinse using one cup of vinegar and two cups of water. Be sure to close your eyes tightly when using. Your hair will be squeaky clean.

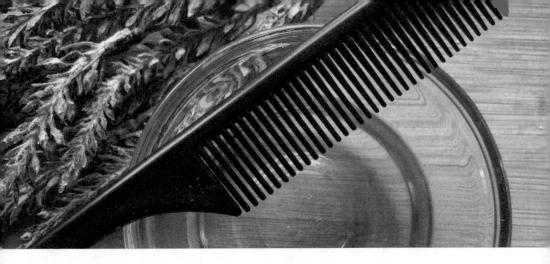

Scented Hair Rinse

Make your own scented hair rinse by adding herbs and spices to white vinegar. Let the vinegar sit for two weeks before using. Strain the rinse and store in a spray bottle. Use after shampooing and rinse. Your hair will look and smell clean and fresh.

Head Lice Treatment

If you or someone you know has head lice, rinse hair in vinegar before using a lice treatment. This will help to loosen nits from the hair shaft.

Hairbrush Cleaner

Clean your hairbrush and comb by soaking them in a sink full of hot water with one cup of white vinegar.

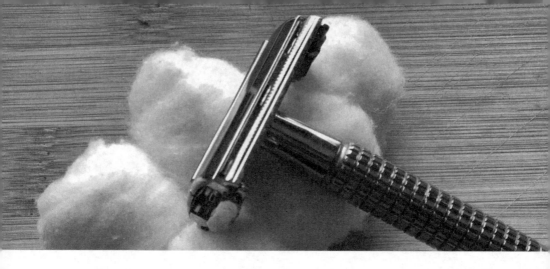

Aftershave Treatment

Undiluted vinegar makes an excellent aftershave treatment.

Face Toner

Use equal parts vinegar and water with a few drops of tea tree essential oil for an effective and cost friendly face toner.

Facial Steam

Create a spa-like facial steaming experience at home. Pour boiling water into a large bowl along with some nutmeg and oregano. Lower your face over the bowl and cover your head with a towel. Be careful not to burn your face. Hang over the bowl for a few minutes. Dab your face with a cotton ball soaked in apple cider vinegar to remove dirt and oil from your skin. After your face is cooled, dab more vinegar on your skin to close pores.

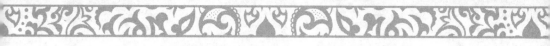

More beauty uses for vinegar

- Wrap your feet in a cloth soaked in vinegar to soften your skin before a pedicure.

- Use full strength vinegar to lighten freckles on your body.

- Mix equal parts onion juice and vinegar, then apply to skin to reduce age spots. This won't work overnight, but over time you will see a huge difference.

- To reduce muscle soreness, soak in a warm tub with one cup of vinegar and 1/4 cup Epsom salt.

- Use white vinegar as a natural deodorant. Spray or splash it on for all-day freshness.

- Brush your teeth once or twice a week with a mixture of white vinegar and baking soda. This will help whiten your teeth and kill bacteria.

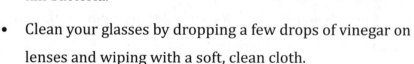

- Clean your glasses by dropping a few drops of vinegar on lenses and wiping with a soft, clean cloth.

- To make your nail polish last longer, wipe nails with a cotton ball dipped in vinegar before painting.

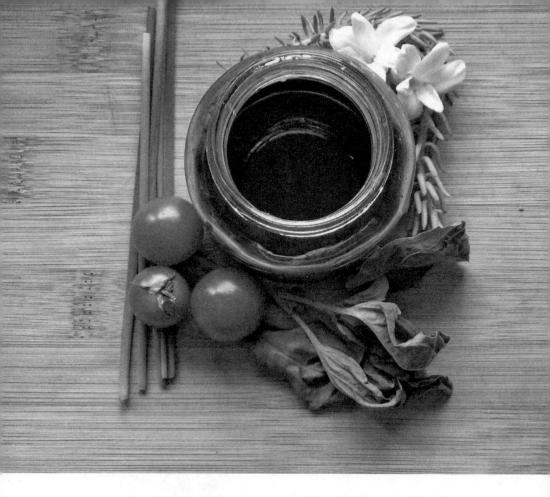

Vinegar in the Kitchen

As mentioned earlier, vinegar is no stranger to the kitchen. In fact, vinegar has often been regarded as one of the most important kitchen staples ever. Here are just some of the ways to use vinegar in your kitchen.

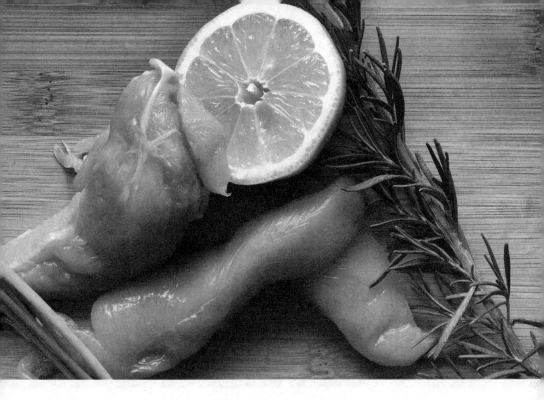

Using vinegar with meat, poultry and fish

Because of its tenderizing capabilities, you can use vinegar in meat marinades. It helps to soften meat and is a great addition to any slow cooked meat meal.

Marinating and basting with vinegar

Less tender cuts of meat such as flank steak benefit greatly from a few hours soaking in a vinegar-based marinade. Basting meat while it cooks on the grill or in the oven is a great way to enhance flavor and keep the meat tender.

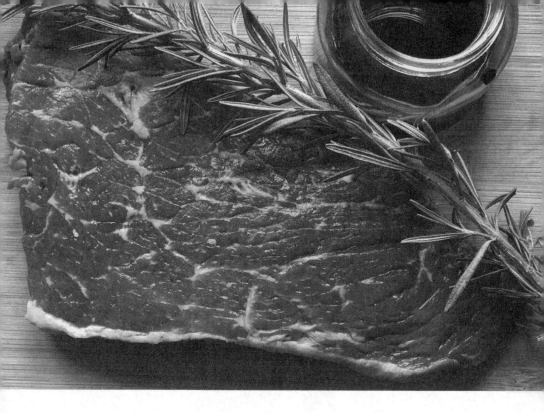

Basic Vinegar Meat Marinade

- ☑ 1/2 cup white or rice vinegar
- ☑ 1/4 cup avocado oil
- ☑ 1/4 cup organic ketchup (or homemade)
- ☑ 1 cup coconut crystals
- ☑ 5 tbsp liquid aminos

Mix all of the ingredients together in a glass jar and shake well.

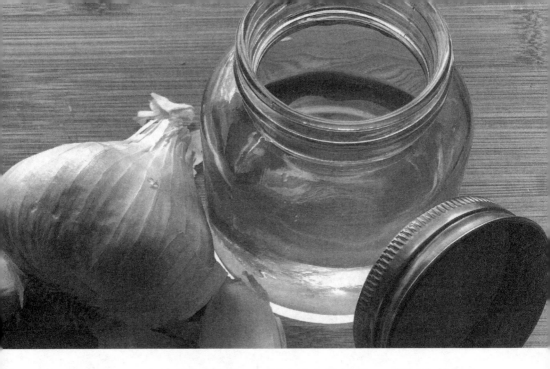

Basic Vinegar Basting Sauce

- ☑ 1/2 cup coconut crystals
- ☑ 1/4 cup rice vinegar
- ☑ 1/4 cup organic ketchup (or homemade)
- ☑ 2 tbsp liquid aminos
- ☑ 2 crushed garlic cloves
- ☑ 2 cloves garlic, crushed
- ☑ 2 tbsp arrowroot

Place all ingredients in a saucepan and heat on medium heat until well mixed.

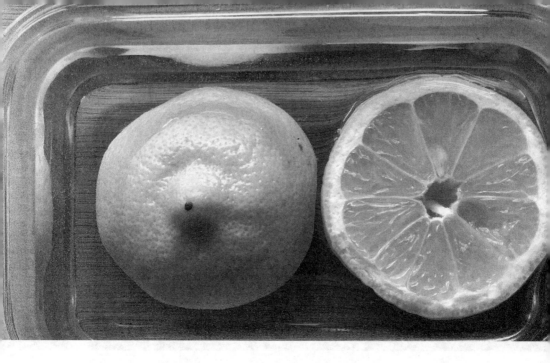

Other ways to use vinegar with meat, poultry and fish

- **Kill bacteria:** Kill bacteria on meat, poultry and fish using a vinegar wash prior to cooking. Mix 2/3 cup lemon juice with 1 cup white vinegar and pour over meat, poultry or fish. Soak for 15 minutes. Pat dry and prepare. If you are cooking a whole chicken, add three tablespoons of the wash to the inside cavity of the chicken and rub on cavity walls. Immerse the chicken at least halfway in the vinegar and lemon wash. Turn the chicken once during the soaking period.

- **Prevent mold:** To prevent mold on the uncooked end of ham, rub vinegar over the area.

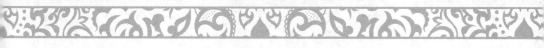

- **Improve taste of boiled ham:** To improve the taste of boiled ham and reduce saltiness, add two tablespoons cider or white vinegar to the water.

- **Tenderize stew meat:** For tender stew meat, add a tablespoon of vinegar while boiling.

- **Scaling fish:** Rubbing fish with vinegar will help make the scaling process easier.

- **Season fish:** Use herbal flavored vinegars to season fish.

- **Poaching:** Add a tablespoon of white vinegar and a tablespoon of sherry to skillet to make poached fish tastier.

Fish Sauce

This fish sauce is a delicious addition to any fish dish.

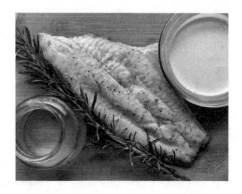

- ☑ 2 tsp white vinegar
- ☑ 1/2 cup heavy cream

Mix ingredients together and pour over cooked fish.

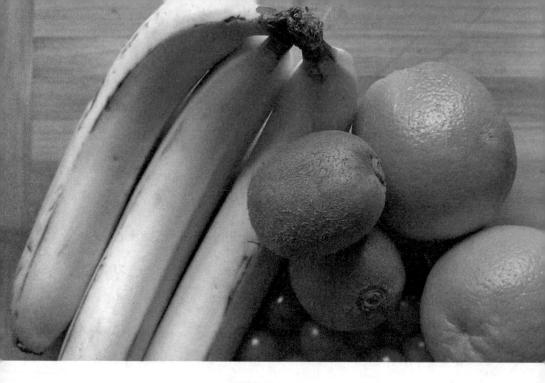

Vinegar for Fruits and Veggies

There are all sorts of fun and tasty ways to use vinegar with fruits and veggies. Here are a few of our favorites:

- Drizzle balsamic or rice vinegar over fresh fruit such as cantaloupe, pears and honeydew. Enjoy immediately.

- Improve the flavor of cooked fruit by adding a teaspoon or two of vinegar while cooking.

- Make a quick and tasty fruit dip by combining a few tablespoons of fruit vinegar with a cup of organic vanilla yogurt.

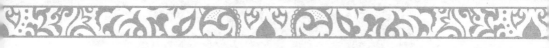

- Replace commercial fruit and veggie wash with a solution of one cup vinegar in a sink half filled with water along with a dash of salt. This will effectively get rid of any bugs in produce.

- Add a spoonful of vinegar to a sink water and soak wilted veggies. They will perk up immediately.

- Add a teaspoon of vinegar to water when you are boiling beets, cauliflower or other veggies. The vinegar will help the vegetables retain their vibrant color, improve their taste and reduce the gassy effects. You can also do this with beans.

- Keep olives and pimentos for a very, very long time by covering with vinegar.

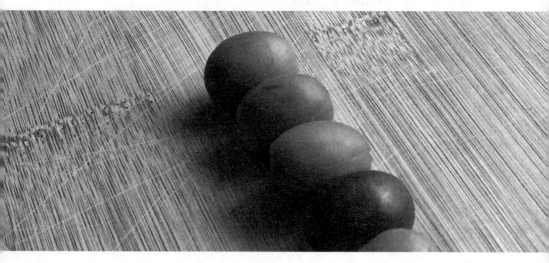

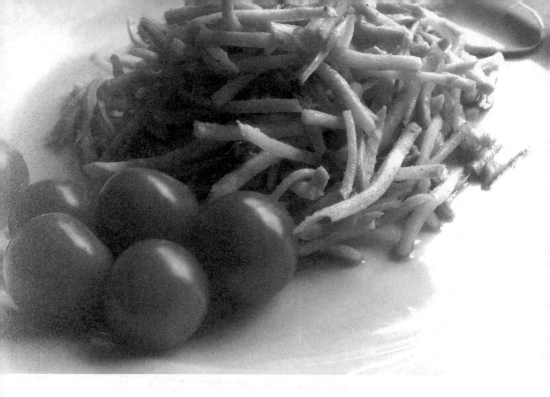

Non-Creamy Coleslaw Dressing

This delicious dressing is low in calories but very tasty.

- ☑ 1 tbsp melted coconut oil
- ☑ 2 tbsp coconut crystals
- ☑ 1/4 cup seasoned rice vinegar
- ☑ 1/2 tsp dry mustard
- ☑ Sea salt and pepper to taste

Mix all ingredients and add to coleslaw.

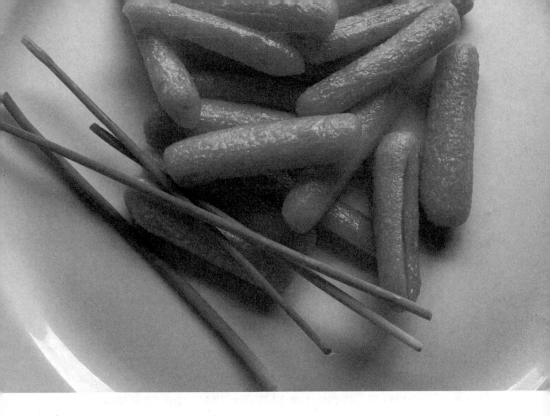

Cooked Veggie Marinade

- ☑ 1 cup coconut crystals
- ☑ 1 cup vinegar
- ☑ 1 cup avocado oil
- ☑ Sea salt and pepper to taste

Heat this mixture on the stovetop on low until blended. Pour over cooked veggies or three bean salad.

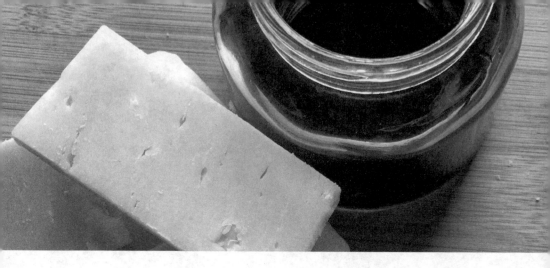

Vinegar and Dairy

Here are some ways to use vinegar with dairy.

- Keep your cheese fresh longer by wrapping it in a cotton cloth moistened with vinegar.

- Add a zesty flavor to white sauce by adding 1/2 teaspoon of your favorite vinegar.

Low-Fat Sour Cream Substitute

- ☑ 12-ounce container small curd cottage cheese
- ☑ 1/4 cup skim milk
- ☑ 2 tsp vinegar
- ☑ 2 tsp coconut sugar

Blend all ingredients together in a food processor.

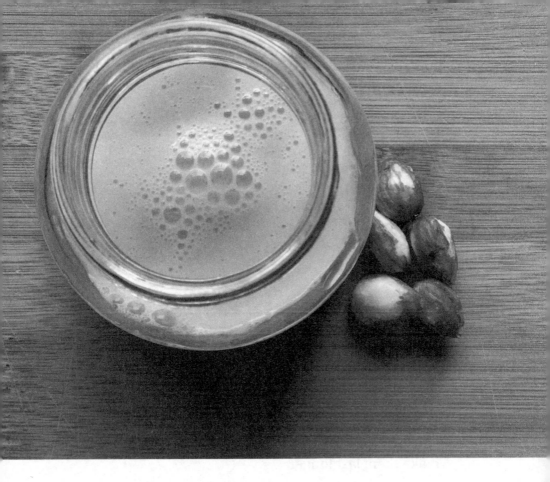

Buttermilk Substitute

- ☑ 1 cup organic milk
- ☑ 1 tbsp vinegar

Add the vinegar to the milk and let it stand until it becomes thick (about 10 minutes).

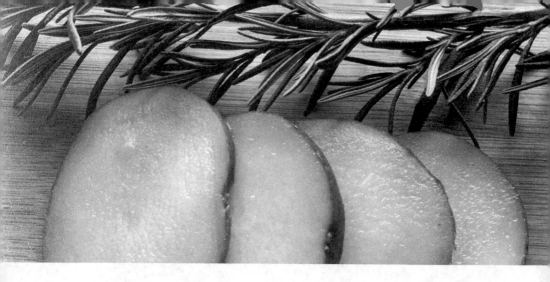

More Ways to Use Vinegar In the Kitchen

- Use malt vinegar in place of ketchup on fries.

- Add a little vinegar to ketchup and other condiments to make them last longer.

- Make your pasta less sticky by adding a dash of vinegar to the cooking water.

- Add a teaspoon of vinegar to your rice water to keep rice from sticking.

- Cover peeled potatoes with water and a dash of vinegar to keep them from discoloring. Be sure to keep them in the refrigerator.

- To give your homemade bread a shiny crust, brush the top with vinegar 10 minutes before baking is finished.

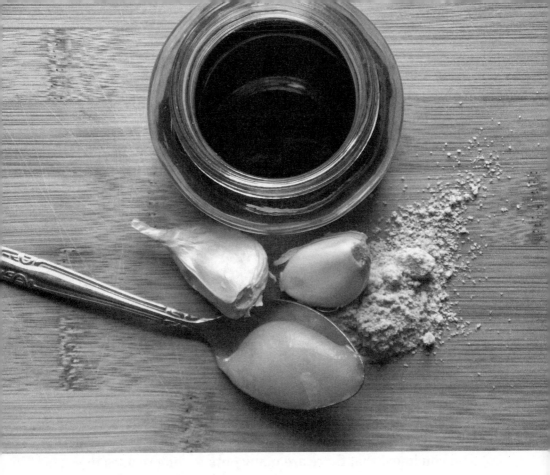

Homemade Garlic Mustard

- ☑ 4 tbsp dry mustard
- ☑ 2 tbsp raw honey
- ☑ 1 tbsp flavored vinegar
- ☑ 1/2 tsp crushed garlic
- ☑ Sea salt to taste

Combine all ingredients and heat on low to blend. Add a little arrowroot if you need to thicken the mixture.

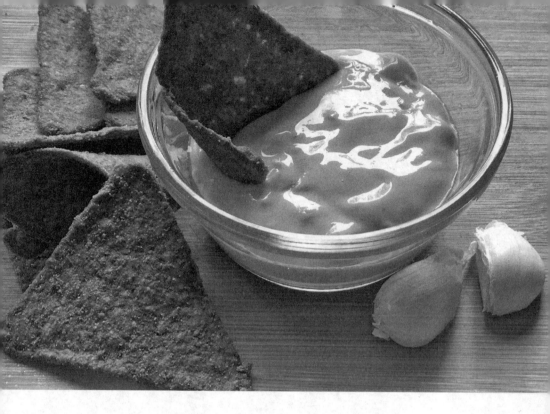

More awesome recipes using vinegar

Did you know that there are many outstanding recipes that can take advantage of the tangy taste and healthful compounds of vinegar? These 17 fantastic recipes will give you another reason to stock up on vinegar.

Vegan Queso Dip

If you're vegan but are really missing that cheesy flavor, or you're planning a party where you need a dip for your vegan guests, this one is sure to be a hit. Using apple cider vinegar in the recipe brings it a sharp edge that's similar to cheddar.

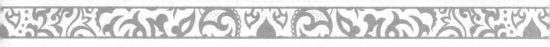

INGREDIENTS

- ☑ 2 tbsp extra virgin olive oil
- ☑ 3 garlic cloves, pressed
- ☑ 1/2 large sweet onion, finely diced
- ☑ 2 large carrots, very finely chopped
- ☑ 1 cup butternut squash, thinly sliced
- ☑ 2 tsp sea salt, divided
- ☑ 1 tsp cumin
- ☑ 1/2 tsp chili powder
- ☑ 1/4 tsp freshly ground black pepper
- ☑ 1 cup vegetable stock
- ☑ 1 1/2 cups unsweetened plain almond milk
- ☑ 1 cup of cashews, soaked for 30 minutes (or overnight) and then drained
- ☑ 1/4 cup nutritional yeast
- ☑ 1/2 cup chunky salsa
- ☑ 1 tbsp apple cider vinegar

OPTIONAL TOPPINGS

- ☑ Pickled jalepeños
- ☑ Chopped cherry tomatoes
- ☑ Cilantro
- ☑ Salsa

INSTRUCTIONS

1. Heat olive oil in a large saucepan over medium heat. Once the oil is hot, add the onions and garlic. Sauté until onions are soft and garlic is fragrant.

2. Add carrots and butternut squash, stir well and then add a teaspoon of the sea salt along with the cumin, chili powder and black pepper. Allow the mixture to cook together for several minutes, then add in the vegetable stock. Let it simmer together, stirring frequently until the veggies are soft and tender.

3. Add vegetables to a high-powered blender, then add the almond milk, cashews, nutritional yeast, chunky salsa, apple cider vinegar and remaining sea salt. Blend together, scraping down the sides as needed. Continue processing until the mixture has reached a thick and creamy consistency.

4. If necessary, adjust seasoning to suit your preference.

5. Once the dip has sufficiently cooled, place it into a pan and then gently warm over low heat to desired temperature.

6. Serve in a bowl and add garnishes if desired.

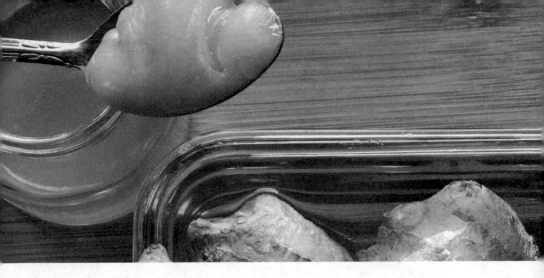

Digestion Soothing Mocktail

This "mocktail" is ideal when you're experience stomach upset and other digestive woes.

INGREDIENTS

- ☑ 2 tsp apple cider vinegar
- ☑ 1 tbsp fresh ginger water (boil fresh ginger root in water, cool and strain liquid)
- ☑ 1 tbsp fresh-squeezed lemon juice
- ☑ 8 ounces sparkling water
- ☑ Raw honey to taste (optional)

INSTRUCTIONS

Combine all ingredients thoroughly. Pour over ice and enjoy.

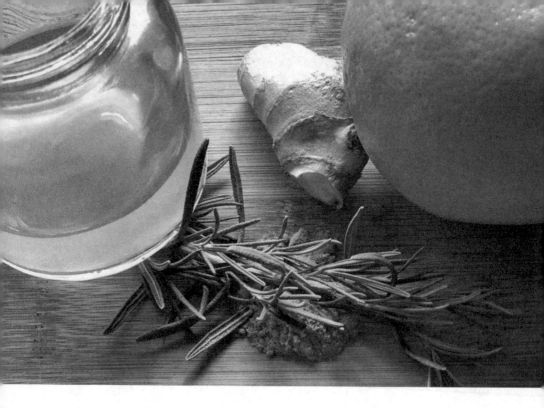

After-Dinner Turmeric Apple Cider Spritzer

This recipe combines two of the hottest superfoods around: turmeric and apple cider vinegar. It's ideal as an after-dinner drink, particularly following a rich meal, as it will help settle your stomach. The herbs and ginger create a fabulous flavor base, with each herb helping to trigger the digestive process. The combination of orange juice and vinegar tempers the stronger herb flavors as well as taking advantage of ACV's ability to soothe digestive woes.

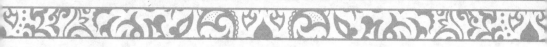

INGREDIENTS

- ☑ 3 sage leaves
- ☑ 1 sprig mint
- ☑ 1 sprig rosemary
- ☑ 1-inch fresh ginger root
- ☑ 1/4 tsp turmeric powder
- ☑ Juice of 1 medium orange
- ☑ 1 cup sparkling water
- ☑ 1 tbsp apple cider vinegar
- ☑ 1 tbsp raw honey
- ☑ 1 to 2 tsp aromatic bitters

INSTRUCTIONS

Combine the first five ingredients in a glass, then stir in the remaining ingredients until thoroughly combined. Strain and serve over ice.

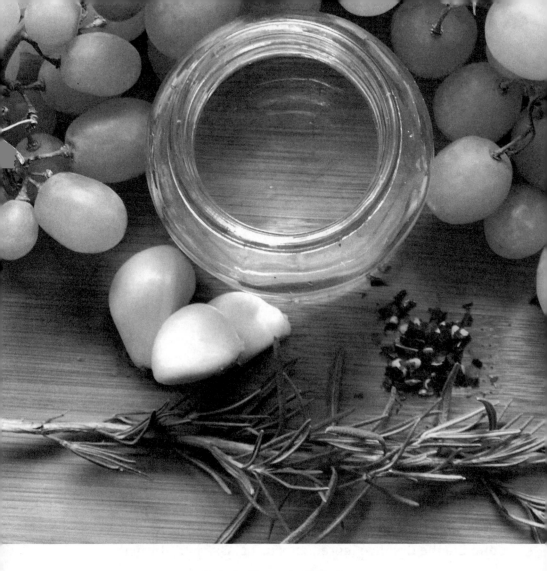

Rosemary and Chile Pickled Grapes

These spicy-tart grapes are ideal for adding to a cheese plate or an antipasto platter thanks to the complex flavors, due in part to the white wine vinegar. And, even better, it only takes 10 minutes to put together.

INGREDIENTS

- ☑ 3 cups seedless green grapes
- ☑ 3 cups seedless red grapes
- ☑ 6 fresh rosemary sprigs (about 4 inches in length), divided
- ☑ 2 cups white wine vinegar
- ☑ 3 garlic cloves, thinly sliced
- ☑ 2 tbsp sea salt
- ☑ 2 tsp raw honey
- ☑ 1/2 tsp dried crushed red pepper
- ☑ 1 cup water

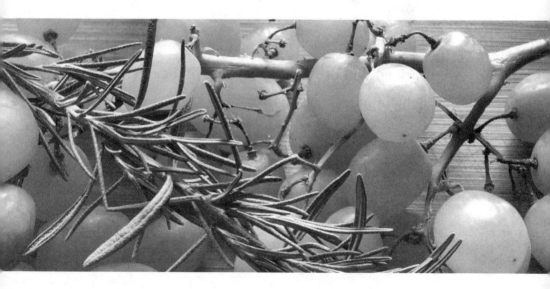

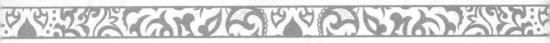

INSTRUCTIONS

1. Add grapes evenly into four pint-sized lidded canning jars.

2. Add one rosemary sprig to each jar.

3. Add white wine vinegar, garlic, sea salt, honey, red pepper, water and two remaining rosemary sprigs to a medium saucepan. Bring the mixture to a simmer, then remove from heat and remove rosemary sprigs.

4. Pour hot vinegar mixture over the grapes and cover loosely. Allow it to cool to room temperature, about 30 minutes.

5. After the mixture has reached room temperature, seal each jar with a lid and then place in the refrigerator to chill for at least an hour.

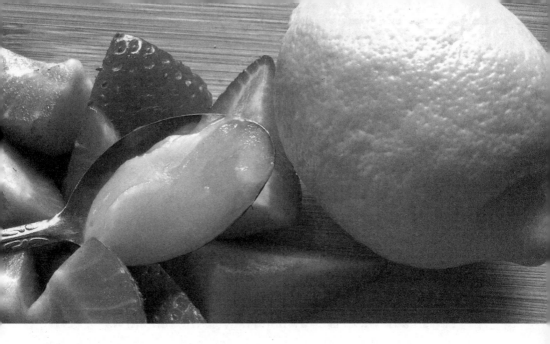

Iced Strawberries With Buttermilk and Balsamic Vinegar

Vinegar can be used to make some fantastic desserts, too, like this granita-style frozen dessert featuring strawberries, lemon juice, buttermilk and balsamic vinegar.

INGREDIENTS

- ☑ 1 tsp raw honey
- ☑ 1 1/2 tbsp fresh-squeezed lemon juice
- ☑ 1 cup buttermilk
- ☑ 1 cup strawberries, cut into quarters

- ☑ 1/2 tsp finely grated lemon zest
- ☑ 1 tsp aged balsamic vinegar
- ☑ 4 small tarragon sprigs, optional

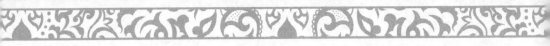

1. Whisk together honey and the 1/2 tablespoon of lemon juice. Whisk in buttermilk and then pour the mixture into a shallow baking dish. Freeze until firm, whisking every half hour for three hours.

2. In a bowl, toss strawberries with the remaining tablespoon of lemon juice and then add lemon juice and balsamic vinegar. Allow to stand for 30 minutes.

3. Spoon berries, along with any juices, into serving glasses.

4. Use a fork to scrape buttermilk ice into fluffy crystals and spoon over strawberries.

5. Garnish with tarragon, if desired, and serve.

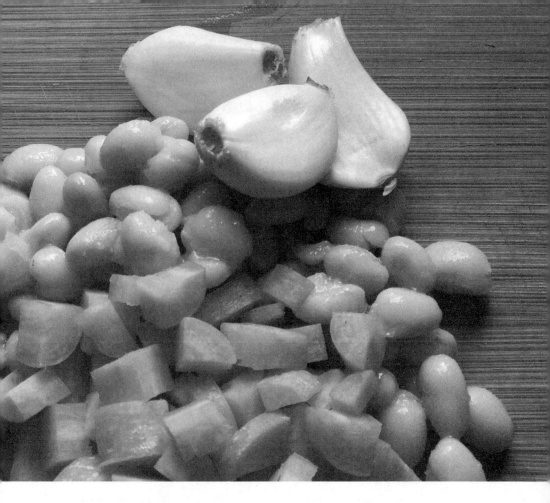

Slow-Cooked Apple Cider Beans

This is a great side dish that goes especially well with a summer BBQ or picnic, particularly when burgers, or veggie burgers, are served. While it takes a while to make, it's definitely worth your time.

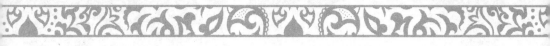

INGREDIENTS

- ☑ 1 pound dry Great Northern beans, soaked overnight
- ☑ 2 tbsp extra virgin olive oil
- ☑ 2 medium sweet onions, diced into small pieces
- ☑ 1 large carrot, diced into small pieces to make about 3/4 cup
- ☑ 1/3 cup tomato paste
- ☑ 3 tbsp blackstrap molasses
- ☑ 1 1/2 tsp Dijon mustard
- ☑ 2 tbsp brown sugar
- ☑ 2 tbsp apple cider vinegar
- ☑ 1 1/2 cups apple cider
- ☑ 1 tsp sea salt
- ☑ 1/4 tsp freshly ground black pepper
- ☑ 2 tsp fresh thyme leaves
- ☑ 4 garlic cloves, minced

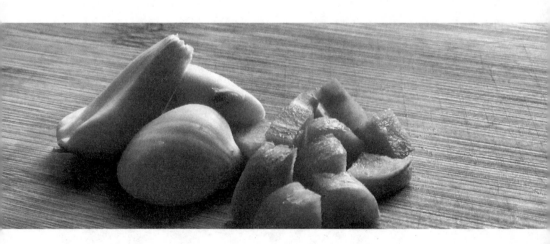

1. Place soaked beans into a medium saucepan over medium-high heat. Add four cups of water, or enough to cover the surface of the beans by about an inch, then bring the liquid to a boil. As soon as it boils, reduce the heat to medium-low and simmer the beans for an hour and a half, until beans are tender.

2. While the beans are cooking, heat the olive oil in a large Dutch oven or saucepan over medium heat. When it's hot, add the onions and carrots and cook for 30 minutes until the onions take on a slight orange hue from the carrots. Stir occasionally and don't allow them to brown.

3. Make the base for the cider sauce while the beans and vegetables are cooking by whisking together tomato paste, molasses, mustard and brown sugar until everything is well mixed and smooth. Slowly add vinegar and whisk again until it becomes a loose paste. Pour cider into the paste, whisking continuously to make a fluid mixture. Add salt, pepper and thyme and stir again, then set aside.

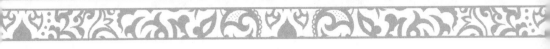

4. Once vegetables have cooked for 30 minutes, add garlic and cook for another two minutes. Add the cider sauce into the pot with the vegetables and mix everything together.

5. When the beans are tender, strain and reserve the cooking liquid. Add the beans to the pot with the cider sauce and then measure 1 1/2 cups of the cooking liquid and add it to the cider sauce. If you don't have enough liquid, add water to make 1 1/2 cups.

6. Simmer the beans in the liquid for 30 to 45 minutes, or until a thicker texture is achieved. You'll get a richer sauce by simmering for at least 45 minutes. Stir occasionally and taste so that seasoning can be adjusted by adding more salt and pepper.

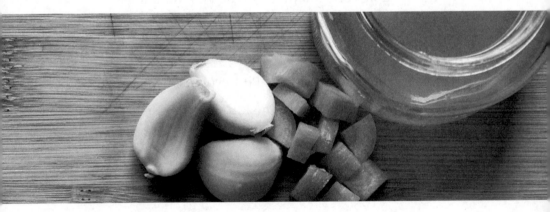

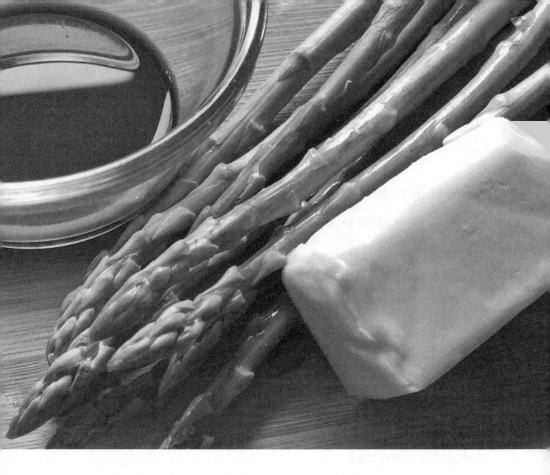

Penne with Roasted Asparagus and Balsamic Butter

In this recipe, balsamic vinegar is used to create a thick, sweet glaze that can be tossed with asparagus or any vegetable that's in season, along with grass-fed butter and pasta. It's incredibly simple to substitute seasonal veggies, like roasted bell pepper strips or green beans for the asparagus. When hot pasta and butter is tossed with the glaze, you'll get a smooth sauce with a fabulous unique flavor.

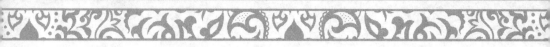

INGREDIENTS

- ☑ 1 lb asparagus
- ☑ 1 tbsp extra virgin olive oil
- ☑ 2 tsp sea salt
- ☑ 1/2 tsp freshly ground black pepper
- ☑ 1/2 cup plus 2 tbsp balsamic vinegar
- ☑ 1/2 tsp brown sugar
- ☑ 1 pound penne
- ☑ 1/4 pound grass-fed butter, cut into pieces
- ☑ 1/3 cup freshly grated Parmesan cheese, plus more for serving

INSTRUCTIONS

1. Preheat the oven to 400°F.

2. In the meantime, snap tough ends off asparagus and discard them. Cut them into approximately 1-inch spears. Place asparagus on a baking sheet and toss with the oil and 1/4 teaspoon each of the sea salt and pepper. Roast until tender, about 10 minutes.

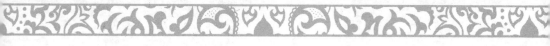

3. Place balsamic vinegar into a small saucepan. Simmer until three tablespoons remain. Stir in brown sugar and remaining 1/4 teaspoon pepper. Remove from the heat.

4. Cook penne in large pot of boiling water until just done, about 13 minutes. Drain pasta and toss with butter, vinegar, asparagus, Parmesan cheese and remaining sea salt.

5. Serve with additional Parmesan cheese.

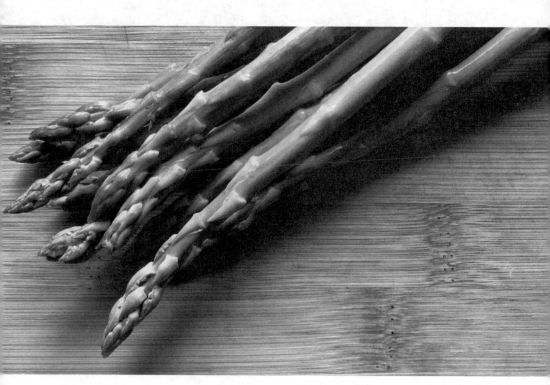

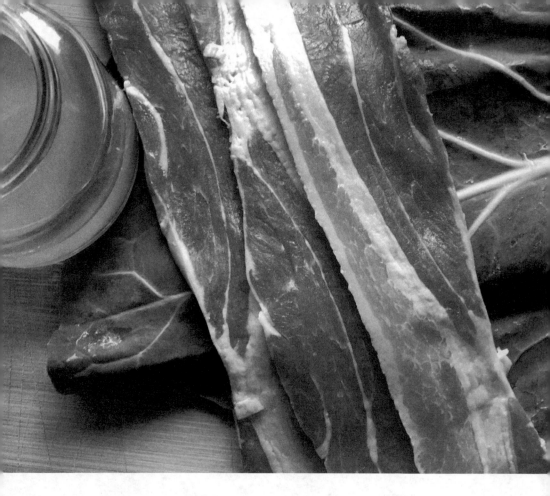

Kimchi and Collard Greens

This dish is an ideal mix of kimchi and collard greens. While it may not seem like a mash-up that would work, it's surprisingly yummy with the combination of spicy Korean fermented veggies and classic southern comfort.

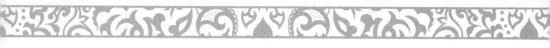

INGREDIENTS

- ☑ 1 tbsp extra virgin olive oil
- ☑ 5 slices thick-cut (free-range organic) bacon, cut into 1-inch pieces
- ☑ 1/2 medium sweet onion, peeled and diced
- ☑ 2 bunches collard greens
- ☑ 2 tbsp apple cider vinegar
- ☑ 1 cup chicken or vegetable broth
- ☑ 1 14-ounce jar kimchi

INSTRUCTIONS

1. Cook the bacon by heating the oil in a large skillet (not nonstick) over medium-high heat until it shimmers. Add chopped bacon and cook until crisp around the edges, stirring occasionally with a wooden spoon. Remove bacon to a plate that's been lined with paper towels, then set aside. With bacon grease still in the skillet, add onion and sauté until softened, translucent and just about caramelized, from 8 to 10 minutes.

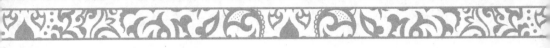

2. Prepare collard greens while the onion and bacon are cooking. Stack a few of the leaves onto a cutting board and cut off the stems. Cut the leaves crosswise into long, 1-inch wide strips, then cut the strips into 2-inch pieces. Repeat with remaining collard leaves. Place collards into a colander and rinse under running water; gently shake to remove excess water. When onion is nearly caramelized, add collards, one handful at a time. Heat and stir until collards begin to cook down, about two minutes, then add another handful of collards. Repeat until all collards are added to the skillet.

3. Deglaze the pan by pushing the collards to one side of the skillet, exposing the browned bits at the bottom. Add vinegar and stir immediately. Add broth, reduce heat to medium and continue to cook, stirring occasionally until nearly all liquid has evaporated, about 10 to 15 minutes.

4. Once the liquid has just about evaporated and what remains is golden brown and thick, remove the skillet from the heat. Add kimchi and stir until thoroughly mixed. Transfer to a serving dish and top with the crisp bacon pieces.

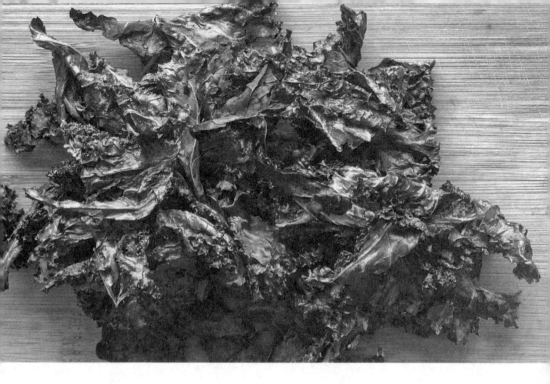

Sea Salt and Vinegar Kale Chips

If you're looking for a healthy, savory snack, it's hard to beat this kale chip recipe. This classic combination is irresistible, yet there's really no reason to feel guilty about indulging. And, even better, it's simple to make.

INGREDIENTS

- ☑ 1 bunch Lascinato kale (or curly kale)
- ☑ 2 tbsp apple cider vinegar
- ☑ 1 tbsp extra virgin olive oil
- ☑ 1/2 tsp coarse sea salt

INSTRUCTIONS

1. Preheat oven to 350°F. In the meantime, wash and dry kale leaves.

2. Use a knife to separate kale leaves from the thick ribs, then discard the ribs. Cut or tear the leaves into your desired size of chips, keeping in mind that they will shrink a little while baking.

3. Combine kale leaves, vinegar, olive oil and sea salt in a large bowl. Use your hands to toss the kale for a couple of minutes, until it turns slightly darker and soft.

4. Spread out the kale in a single layer onto a baking sheet covered with parchment paper.

5. Sprinkle on remaining salt, and bake for 7 to 10 minutes, until kale is crunchy.

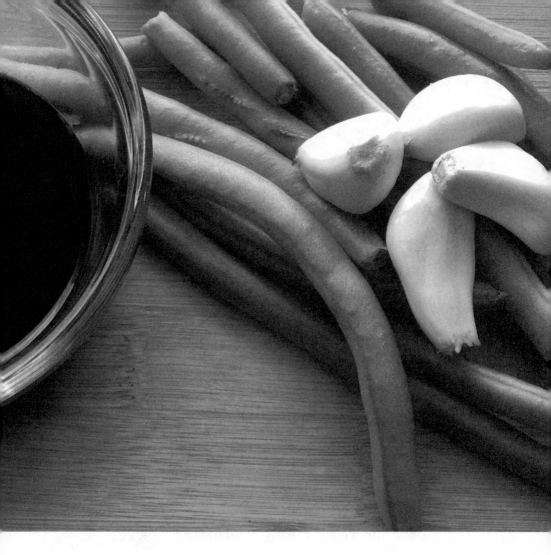

Balsamic Green Beans With Walnuts

This is a wonderfully healthy, seasonal recipe that's ideal if you have picky kids who don't like to eat their vegetables. In fact, you might even be surprised to find them coming back for more.

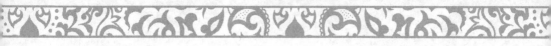

INGREDIENTS

- ☑ 4 tsp extra virgin olive oil
- ☑ 4 tsp garlic, minced
- ☑ 1/2 cup chopped walnuts, toasted
- ☑ 2 tsp aged balsamic vinegar
- ☑ 1/2 tsp sea salt
- ☑ 1 pound green beans, trimmed

INSTRUCTIONS

1. Heat oil in a small skillet over medium heat. Add garlic and cook, stirring until the garlic just starts to look like it will turn brown, about 30 to 90 seconds. Immediately pour into a large mixing bowl to stop cooking.

2. Add one to two inches of water to a large pot fitted with a steamer attachment, cover and bring to a boil over high heat. Add green beans to steamer and cook covered until the beans are crisp tender, four to five minutes.

3. Transfer the green beans to the bowl. Add walnuts, balsamic and salt. Toss to coat.

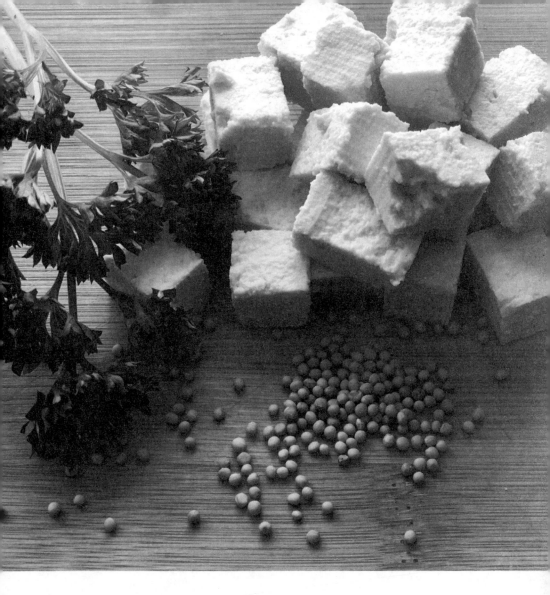

Tangy Curried Tofu Salad

This delicious vegan-friendly curried tofu salad is ideal to pile onto a bed of greens, fill a lettuce wrap or a sandwich.

INGREDIENTS

- ☑ 1/3 cup golden raisins
- ☑ 1 tsp yellow mustard seeds
- ☑ ¼ cup apple cider vinegar
- ☑ 1 lb extra firm tofu
- ☑ 2 tbsp roasted pumpkin seeds
- ☑ 1 scallion, chopped
- ☑ 1 tbsp chopped parsley
- ☑ 1/2 cup vegan mayonnaise
- ☑ 2 tbsp curry powder
- ☑ 3/4 tsp sea salt
- ☑ Freshly ground black pepper

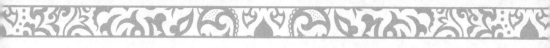

INSTRUCTIONS

1. Add raisins and mustard seeds to a small heatproof bowl. Bring the apple cider vinegar to a boil and pour it over the raisins and mustard seeds. Allow them to soak for at least 10 minutes, the longer the better.

2. Rinse and drain tofu, then press it gently between towels to eliminate excess water. Place the tofu into a large bowl and crumble it roughly with your hands.

3. Add mustard seeds, any remaining vinegar, pumpkin seeds, scallions and parsley.

4. In a separate bowl, stir together vegan mayonnaise, curry powder, sea salt and pepper to taste. Add this to the tofu mixture and stir until well-combined. Taste and adjust seasonings if desired.

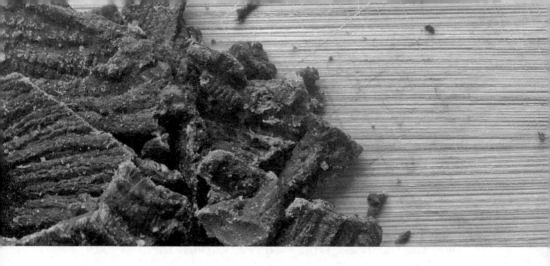

Apple Cider Vinegar Beef Jerky

Not only is beef jerky packed with protein, this recipe calls for apple cider vinegar and kefir, which means you'll get a healthy dose of probiotics too. If you have a dehydrator, you'll definitely want to try it. Even if you don't, it's a great excuse to get one.

INGREDIENTS

- ☑ 1 1/2 pounds sliced grass-fed beef
- ☑ 1 tbsp liquid aminos
- ☑ 1/4 cup apple cider vinegar
- ☑ 1/4 cup water kefir
- ☑ 1 tsp grated fresh ginger root
- ☑ 3 garlic cloves, crushed
- ☑ Juice of 1/2 a lemon
- ☑ 1 tsp Dijon mustard
- ☑ 1 1/2 tbsp coconut sugar
- ☑ Black pepper to taste
- ☑ Coconut oil to grease

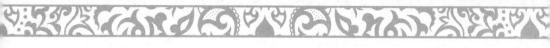

INSTRUCTIONS

1. Prepare the marinade by combining all the ingredients together in a bowl, except the beef and coconut oil. Taste and adjust if necessary.

2. Add the meat to the marinade, cover and allow to sit for 10 to 24 hours.

3. Rub coconut oil onto baking/dehydrator sheets.

4. Cut beef strips into bite size pieces and place onto the dehydrator sheets.

5. Dehydrate at 113°F, which helps retain the probiotics in the kefir and apple cider vinegar.

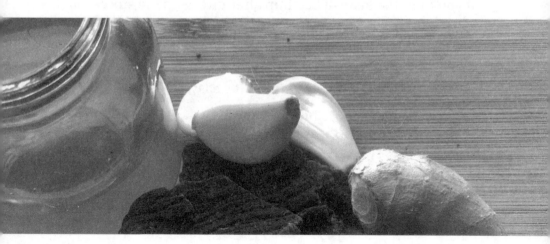

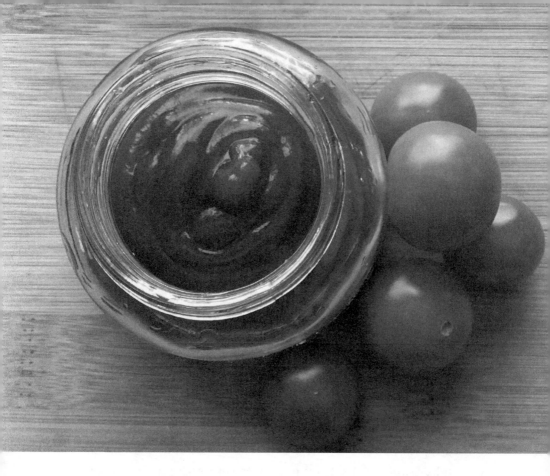

Healthy Homemade Ketchup

If you miss the taste of ketchup after giving up the store-bought stuff (which is typically filled with high fructose corn syrup), you'll be happy to know that you can make your own healthy version using apple cider vinegar. It's easy, takes two minutes to make and it's incredibly tasty too.

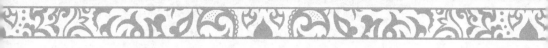

INGREDIENTS

- ☑ 8 oz tomato paste
- ☑ 4 tbsp pure maple syrup
- ☑ 2 tbsp apple cider vinegar
- ☑ 1 tsp onion powder
- ☑ 1 tsp oregano
- ☑ Sea salt to taste

INSTRUCTIONS

Combine all ingredients in a bowl. Taste and adjust seasonings if necessary. That's it!

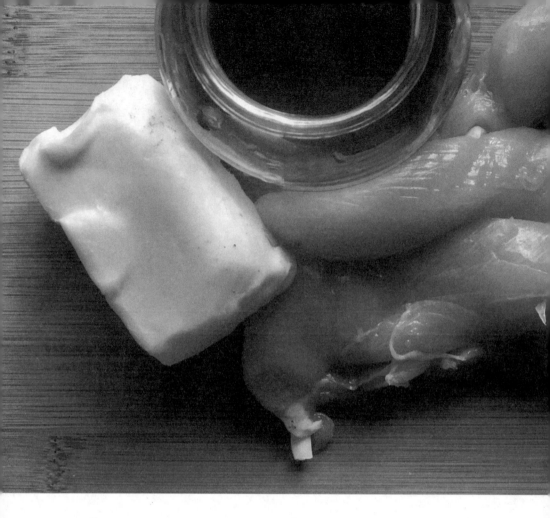

Chicken Sauteed with Red Wine Vinegar

Chicken with vinegar is considered one of the great poultry dishes from the Lyons, France region — known for producing some of the world's best chickens. As the red wine vinegar in that area typically contains five percent acidity, and U.S. wine vinegars are usually seven percent acidity, the recipe adds water to cut strong vinegar.

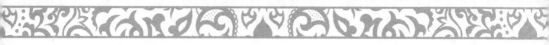

INGREDIENTS

- ☑ 2 tbsp extra virgin olive oil
- ☑ 1 3-lb organic, free-range chicken, cut up for sauteing
- ☑ Sea salt and fresh ground black pepper, to taste
- ☑ 1/4 cup scallions
- ☑ 1 cup high quality red-wine vinegar
- ☑ 1 tbsp grass-fed butter

INSTRUCTIONS

1. Preheat the oven to 450°F. Place a large ovenproof skillet over medium-high heat and add the olive oil. When the oil is hot, add the chicken to the skillet, skin side down. Cook for about five minutes, without disturbing, or until chicken is nicely browned. Turn and cook three minutes on the other side. Season with salt and pepper, to taste.

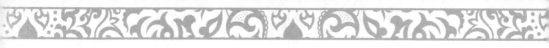

2. Place skillet into the oven and cook for 15 to 20 minutes, until almost done — there should be just a trace of pink near the bone. Remove chicken and place on an ovenproof platter. Put it in the oven and then turn off the heat, leaving the door slightly ajar.

3. Pour all but two tablespoons of the cooking juices out of the skillet and discard. Place skillet over medium-high heat and add scallions, sprinkling them with a little salt and pepper. Cook, stirring until tender, about two minutes.

4. Add vinegar and raise the heat to high. Cook a minute or two, or until the strong acrid smell has subsided a bit. Add 1/2 cup water and cook for another two minutes, stirring until the mixture is slightly reduced and somewhat thickened. Stir in butter.

5. Return the chicken and any accumulated juices to the skillet, then turn the chicken in the sauce.

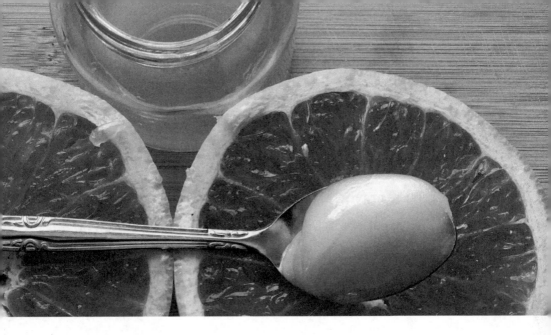

Pink Energy-Boosting Super Juice

If you're looking for a refreshing juice that will start your day off with a burst of energy, this is it! Plus, it takes just seconds to put together so you can even make it on your busiest mornings.

INGREDIENTS

- ☑ 1 1/2 cups fresh pink grapefruit juice
- ☑ 1 to 2 tbsp apple cider vinegar
- ☑ 2 tsp raw honey

INSTRUCTIONS

Mix all ingredients in a tall glass and enjoy, with or without ice.

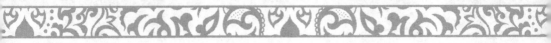

Salt and Vinegar Roasted Potatoes

When you're craving the taste of salt and vinegar chips and kale chips just won't cut it, this is a great alternative. You can jazz things up even more by tossing in fresh herbs for more flavor and nutrition.

INGREDIENTS

- ☑ 2 lbs small red potatoes
- ☑ 2 tbsp extra virgin olive oil
- ☑ 3 tbsp apple cider vinegar, divided (white and red wine vinegar can also be used)
- ☑ 1 tsp sea salt, divided
- ☑ 1/4 tsp fresh ground black pepper

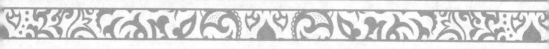

INSTRUCTIONS

1. Preheat oven to 400°F. In the meantime, cut up red potatoes into approximately 1 1/2-inch chunks.

2. In a large bowl, add olive oil, vinegar and 1/2 teaspoon each of sea salt and pepper. Stir to evenly coat potatoes.

3. Place potatoes onto a large baking sheet, spreading into an even layer, and cook for 25 minutes.

4. Use a spatula to scrape up potatoes from the baking sheet and flip over. Cook for another 20 minutes, then repeat with the spatula to scrape potatoes.

5. Drizzle potatoes with another tablespoon of vinegar and the remaining 1/2 teaspoon of sea salt. Stir potatoes to evenly coat.

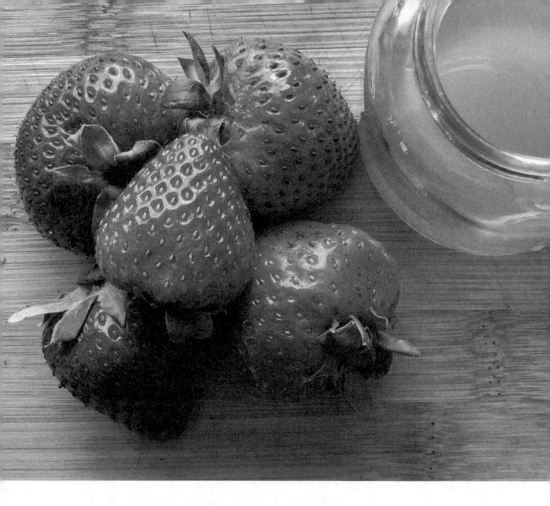

Berries with Apple Cider Vinegar and Cashew Cream Breakfast Bowl

This amazing breakfast bowl could also be made as a wonderful dessert. It's so good, it's hard to believe that it's actually good for you too.

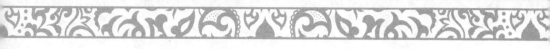

INGREDIENTS

- ☑ 2 cups fresh berries (you can use a mix such as blueberries, blackberries, strawberries, raspberries, etc.)
- ☑ 4 tsp apple cider vinegar
- ☑ 1/2 cup slivered almonds
- ☑ 1 cup raw cashew nuts
- ☑ 2/3 cup filtered water
- ☑ 8 drops stevia liquid

INSTRUCTIONS

1. Make the cashew nut cream the night before by placing all ingredients into a food processor or high speed blender. Mix until smooth and creamy. Add a little more water if the mixture isn't smooth enough.

2. Divide berries between two small bowls

3. Add two teaspoons of apple cider vinegar to each bowl and then top with slivered almonds and cashew nut cream.

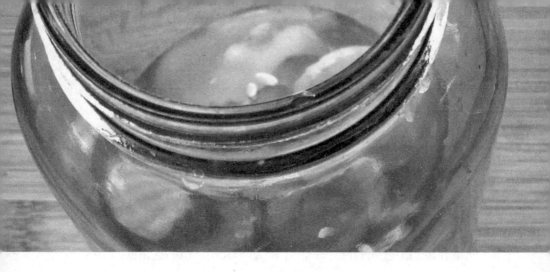

Pickling

Pickling with vinegar has been practiced for centuries and is an age-old method for preserving food. Because of its high acid content, vinegar creates an atmosphere where bacteria can't survive.

Here are some tips for perfect pickling:

- Always use a glass or ceramic container. If you use metal or plastic, it will react with the acid.

- Most recipes call for white distilled vinegar which has a very tart and distinct flavor. It does not change the color of pale veggies or fruits. Apple cider vinegar has a fruity taste and may darken veggies and fruits.

- Do not use flavored vinegars and do not dilute vinegar with water unless the recipe calls for it.

Refrigerator Pickles

The whole family will love these easy-to-make pickles.

- ☑ 1 cup sugar
- ☑ 1 cup hot water
- ☑ 1/2 cup white vinegar
- ☑ 2 cucumbers, sliced thin and in circular fashion

- ☑ Bunch green onions cut into 1-inch pieces
- ☑ Glass mason jar

Pour the sugar into the mason jar and cover with hot water. Stir until the sugar dissolves. Add the white vinegar and stir once more. Add the cucumbers and cover the jar. Allow the jar to set in the refrigerator for at least 12 hours before serving.

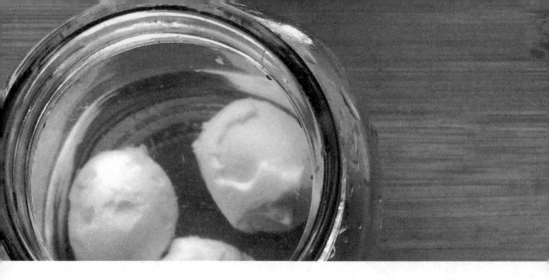

Pickled Eggs

These delicious eggs will keep for two months in the refrigerator.

- ☑ One dozen eggs, hard cooked and peeled
- ☑ 1 small white onion
- ☑ 3 cups white vinegar
- ☑ 3-inch cinnamon stick
- ☑ 1 tbsp raw honey
- ☑ 1 tsp whole allspice
- ☑ 1 tsp whole clove
- ☑ 1/2 tsp coriander seeds
- ☑ Small piece ginger
- ☑ Bay leaf
- ☑ Wide-mouthed mason jar

Place eggs along with onion in the jar. Place the vinegar, cinnamon, honey, spices, coriander, ginger and bay leaf in a saucepan. Bring mixture to a boil and simmer for five minutes. Allow the mixture to cool and pour over the eggs. Place eggs in the refrigerator for a week before eating.

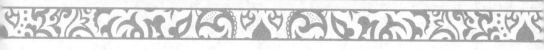

Bust Odors With Vinegar

Not only is vinegar a great compliment to the chef, it can also be used to bust those stubborn odors that often lurk in your kitchen. Here are some tips for how to use it:

- Put a small amount of vinegar in a bowl and leave it in any room to remove odors.

- Rub some vinegar on your hands to remove odors from cooking. It will also remove stains from berries.

- Remove odors by filling a pan halfway with water and adding in 1/4 cup of vinegar and three cinnamon sticks. Allow the mixture to boil and simmer as the steam fills the room.

- If your garbage disposal stinks, try this trick. Fill an ice cube tray up with vinegar and freeze. Put the cubes into the disposal and run for five seconds with water.

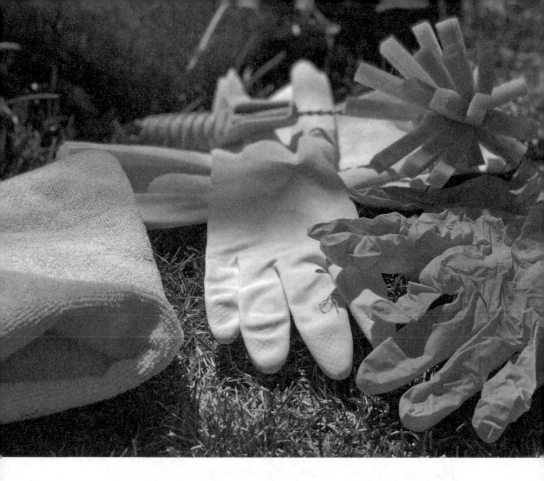

Cleaning and Sanitizing

Just as vinegar can help to bust nasty odors, it can also keep your home sparkling clean. Applying white vinegar to surfaces kills viruses, mold and bacteria, and also discourages them from growing there in the future. Keeping a jug of distilled vinegar on hand in the kitchen for cleaning is a great and economical way to disinfect and deodorize.

Here are just some of the ways to use vinegar for a sparkling kitchen. Note: Unless otherwise mentioned, use white vinegar:

- Remove mineral deposits from fixtures by making a paste from two tablespoons salt and one tablespoon vinegar. Spread paste with a soft cloth and buff.

- Make an all-purpose cleaner by mixing 1/2 cup white vinegar in a spray bottle with two tablespoons for baking soda and a few drops of lemon essential oil. Shake well before using.

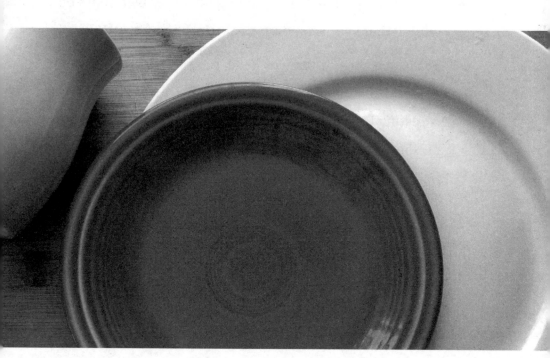

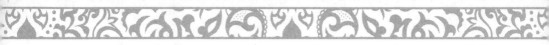

- Sanitize your dishwasher by placing a dishwasher safe cup of white vinegar on the top shelf of the dishwasher and running it on the hot cycle.

- To clean your microwave, boil a solution of 1/4 cup white distilled vinegar and a cup of water in the microwave until you can see steam on the window. The food residue will wipe away easily.

- Clean a vinyl floor with equal parts warm water and vinegar.

- Prevent soap scum from building up on shower doors by wiping them with a sponge soaked in vinegar.

- To clean a clogged shower head, put some vinegar in a plastic bag and wrap it around the shower head so that it is resting in the vinegar. Allow it to set overnight and turn on shower to rinse it off.

- Clean your blinds with a solution made of half white vinegar and half hot water. Dip a white cloth into the solution and wipe the blinds easily.

- To remove rings left on wood furniture, make a solution of vinegar and olive oil and apply it with a soft cloth, going with the grain. Buff with another clean soft cloth.

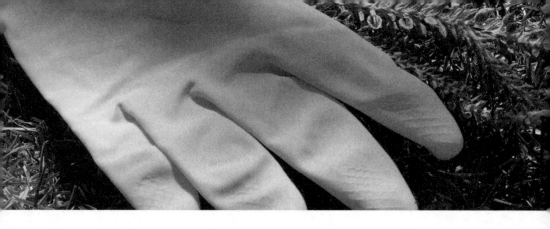

Tips for Removing Carpet Stains

- For light and small carpet stains, make a mixture of two tablespoons salt dissolved in 1/2 cup white vinegar. Allow the solution to dry and then vacuum.

- For stains that are larger or darker, make the same mixture as above but add in two tablespoons of Borax and clean in the same fashion.

- If you have tough, ground in stains, it is best to make a paste with one tablespoon of vinegar and one tablespoon of cornstarch. Rub the mixture into the stain with a dry cloth. Let it set for two days and vacuum.

- For a spray-on spot cleaner, fill a spray bottle with five parts water and one part vinegar and a second spray bottle with one part non-sudsy ammonia and five parts water. Saturate the stain with the first solution and let it set for a few minutes. Blot with a clean, dry cloth. Next, spray and blot using the ammonia solution. Repeat this until the stain is gone.

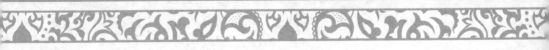

- To give your brick fireplace a facelift, simply go over bricks with a damp cloth soaked in a mixture of one gallon warm water and one cup of vinegar. You can also do this for brick floors.

- To give your leather furniture a boost, mix equal parts vinegar and boiled linseed oil in a spray bottle. Spray the mixture on your furniture and spread it evenly using a soft, clean cloth. Let it set for a minute or two and wipe off with a clean cloth.

- Cut grease on your stovetop by wiping it down with a cloth soaked in vinegar.

- To remove toilet stains, add one gallon of vinegar to the toilet bowl and let it sit. At the same time, saturate a number of paper towels in vinegar and then lay them around the toilet rim to effectively soak the stains. The toilet bowl will end up clean, shiny and disinfected. If stains are very tough, leave the vinegar overnight then sprinkle with baking soda before scrubbing and rinsing.

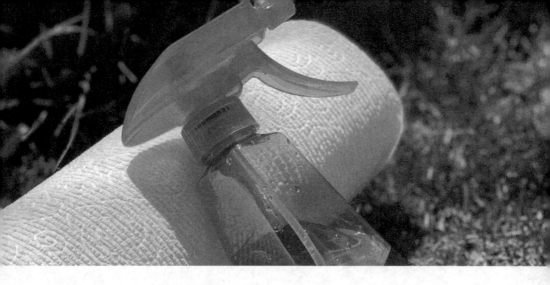

Streak-Free Window Cleaner

Cleaning windows can be a very laborious job. Many commercial cleaners are loaded with dangerous materials and often leave streaks on windows. For a beautiful shine every time, combine 1/3 cup vinegar and 1/3 cup corn starch and apply to windows with a clean cloth. Let the mixture dry and wipe off with a clean, soft cloth.

- Add 1/4 cup of vinegar to your wash cycle to soften fabrics effectively without artificial perfumes and toxins. This simple method also stops static cling!

- If you have trouble with a kitchen drain that smells and harbors drain flies (those tiny brown flies that are more annoying than fruit flies), pour vinegar onto a bottle brush, sprinkle with baking soda and scrub to remove built-up residue in the drain.

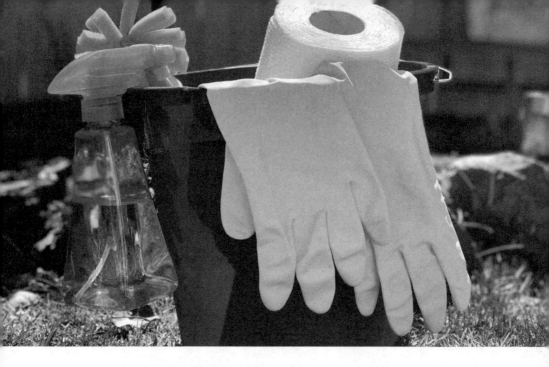

- Use a 50-50 mixture of white vinegar and water to clean windows, the TV or computer screens.

- Heat one cup of vinegar and four tablespoons of baking soda until boiling. Pour into tea and coffee pots to remove mineral buildup.

- Make a solution of equal parts water and vinegar, then spray onto interior surfaces of the refrigerator and wipe dry.

- Use a sponge soaked in vinegar to remove and prevent mildew on your shower curtain.

- Add one tablespoon of vinegar to one cup of water and wipe it over salt stains on footwear. This works best for leather shoes that you can polish afterward.

- Apply vinegar to stickers or glue residue and let it soak in, then scrape off. This works great for bumper stickers.

- Clean and deodorize urine on a mattress using a vinegar and water solution. Sprinkle the affected area with baking soda and let it dry. Brush or vacuum the area after it dries.

- To disinfect and clean wood cutting boards or butcher block countertops, wipe them with full-strength white vinegar each time you use them. As mentioned, acetic acid is a powerful disinfectant and will protect you from harmful bugs such as salmonella, staphylococcus and E. coli. You can also spread some baking soda over the cutting board and cover it in white vinegar to deodorize. Let the foam bubble for five to 10 minutes and rinse with a cloth dipped in cold water.

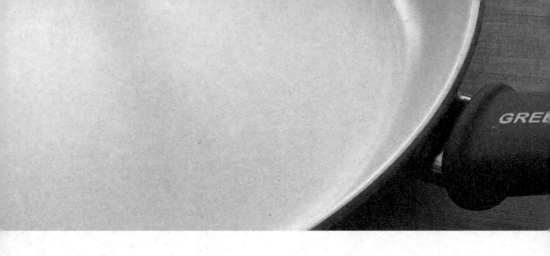

How to clean pots and pans

Combine equal parts of salt and flour in a plastic container.
Add just enough vinegar to make a paste. Spread the paste over
the cooking surface and outside of the pot, then rinse off with
warm water. Dry the pot thoroughly with a soft dish towel.

What not to clean with vinegar

While vinegar is awesome for a vast number of cleaning
jobs, there are some things that don't respond to its acidic
composition, including:

- Granite

- Marble

- Stone floor tiles

- Hardwood floors

- Irons

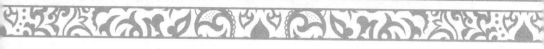

Laundry and Clothes

Here is how to use vinegar for the whitest and brightest clothes.

- To whiten clothes, put a cup of white vinegar in each load along with a 1/4 cup of baking soda. The acid in the vinegar will not harm clothes but is strong enough to dissolve alkalies in detergents and soaps. Vinegar will also help prevent yellowing.

- Adding 1/2 cup vinegar to your wash cycle will help keep static cling at bay.

- When dying fabric, add 1/2 cup vinegar to the last rinse cycle to help set fabric.

- To eliminate manufacturers chemicals from new clothes, wash them with 1/2 cup of vinegar.

**CAUTION: DO NOT USE VINEGAR ON
SILK, RAYONS OR ACETATES**

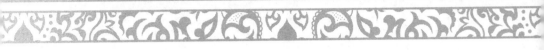

- To make your socks and dishcloths white again, add a cup of vinegar to a large pot of water and bring it to a rolling boil. Drop in items and let them sit overnight.

- To keep bright colors from bleeding in the wash, add one cup of vinegar to a gallon of water and soak items overnight.

- To remove grass stains from clothing, mix water, white vinegar and liquid soap. Scrub on fabric prior to washing.

- Dab some vinegar on mustard stains before washing.

- Make a 50/50 mixture of vinegar and water to pretreat spaghetti, BBQ sauce and ketchup stains.

- Spray full strength vinegar on clothing to remove perspiration stains and odors.

- To fluff up wool and acrylic sweaters, add 1/2 cup white vinegar to final rinse or add when washing by hand.

- Keep table and bed linens from yellowing in storage by adding a cup of vinegar to the rinse cycle.

- Neutralize urine in cloth diapers by adding one cup of vinegar to two gallons of water in the diaper pail. Add another cup of vinegar to the washing machine to further clean and neutralize diapers.

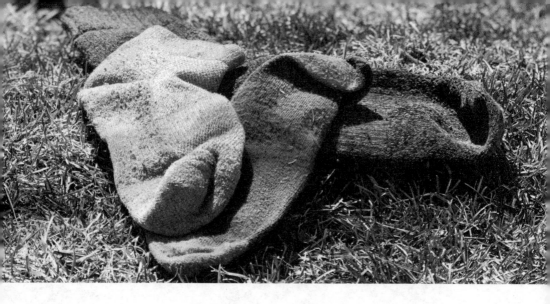

Moldy clothes no more

If you accidentally forgot to change over your laundry and left clothes in the washer too long, simply add a cup of vinegar and wash in hot water. Next, run clothes through a normal cycle and the odor should be gone.

- To remove skunk smell from clothing, add one cup of vinegar to a gallon of water and allow clothes to soak overnight before washing as usual.

- To remove smoke odors from clothing, fill a bathtub full of hot water along with one cup of white vinegar. Hang the clothing over the tub and shut the bathroom door. After a few hours you will notice that the smell is gone.

- Remove crayon stains from clothing by rubbing them with an old toothbrush dipped in vinegar. Wash regularly after rubbing.

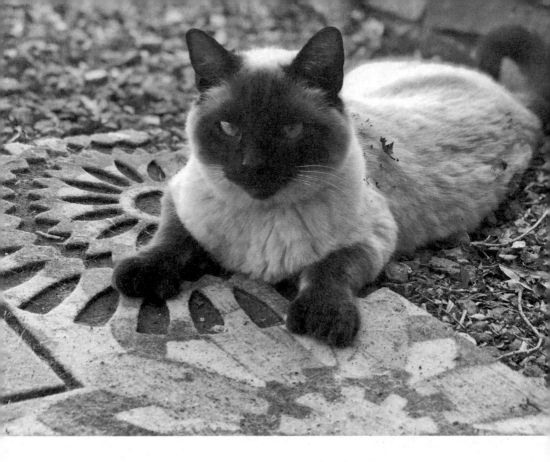

Vinegar and Pets

According to Dr. Judy Morgan, a holistic veterinarian and certified veterinary food therapist from Clayton Veterinary Associates and Churchtown Veterinary Associates in New Jersey, vinegar can be used to treat a number of common health issues found in pets. Not to mention the fact that vinegar is also great for cleaning messes and neutralizing smells associated with animals.

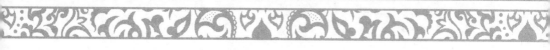

Digestive aid

If you feed your pet a grain-based diet, they may have issues with their digestion because grain will cause a higher-than-healthy level of pH. Adding some vinegar to your pet's food will help them digest it better. In addition, you can try grinding up fresh vegetables and covering them with apple cider vinegar. Let the veggies ferment in the refrigerator a bit and add a bit of this mixture to your pet's food daily.

Keep fleas and ticks at bay

Vinegar will help keep fleas and ticks away from your pets, even your horses. Make a flea and tick repellent by mixing one part vinegar with one part water and spray it on your pet's fur. You can also add a couple of drops of vinegar to your pet's drinking water to help keep fleas and ticks away from the inside out. Generally about one teaspoon per quart of water will work.

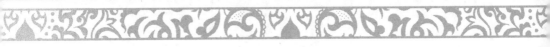

Remedy a urinary tract infection

Before you use vinegar as a remedy for your pet's urinary tract infection, it is important to test your pet's urine pH level. If the pH is above 7, apple cider vinegar can help to lower the pH and dissolve crystals. If the pH is lower than 7, vinegar could make the situation worse. Always check with your veterinarian before using apple cider vinegar for a urinary tract infection.

Hot spots

Organic apple cider vinegar can be an effective treatment for hot spots. It is important to use apple cider vinegar that contains the "mother." The proteins, enzymes and good bacteria will help to ease the pain and inflammation caused by hot spots. Mix equal parts water and vinegar in a spray bottle and spray on hot spots. You can also massage the mixture into the area. Avoid spots that are severely red or open.

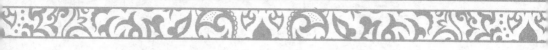

Clean ears

Ear infections are a common occurrence in many dogs, especially those with long and floppy ears. Clean your dog's ears by using a 50/50 mixture of water and vinegar. You can apply the mixture using a cotton ball and wipe the inside of your dog's ears. Remember, only go as far as you can reach. Wiping the ears out with this mixture will change the pH in the ear canal and make it an inhospitable environment for bacteria to grow. If your dog's ears are raw or sore, add more water to the mixture.

Odor buster

One of the most effective ways to get rid of your pet's odor is to spray a thin layer of vinegar over carpet and bedding. Just be careful using vinegar on fabric — always test an area before using.

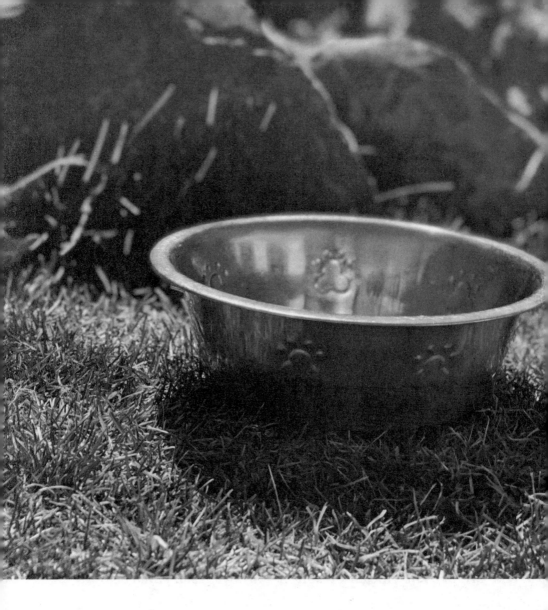

Bowl cleaner

Clean and sanitize your pet's food and water bowls regularly
using a 50/50 mixture of white vinegar and warm water.

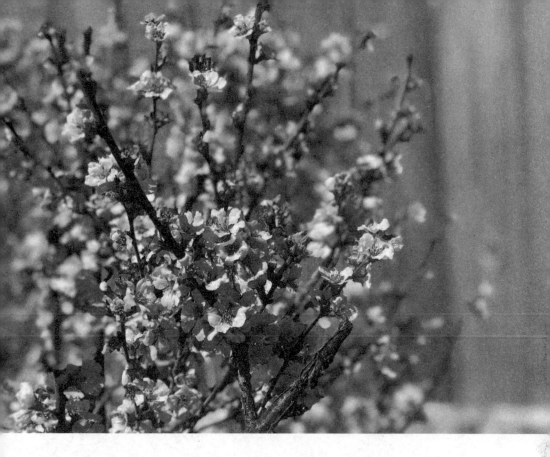

Using Vinegar Outdoors

The benefits of vinegar are not limited to indoor use. Take your jug outside and explore all it can do.

- Acid-loving plants such as azaleas, rhododendrons, hydrangeas and gardenias love a little water from time to time with a vinegar solution. Add one cup of vinegar to a gallon of water and use once a month to keep plants looking their best.

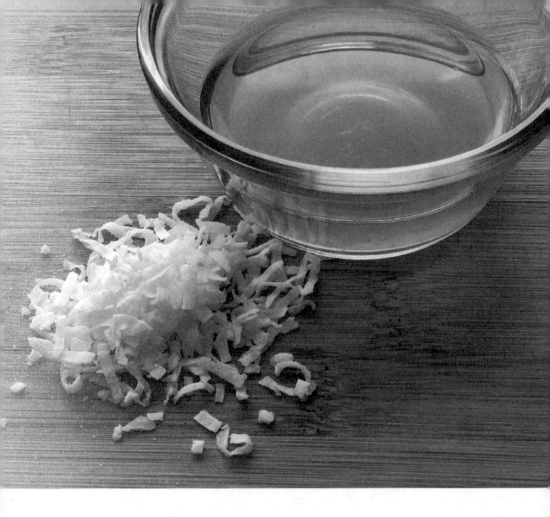

- Pour full strength vinegar on weeds. This is an especially effective treatment for weeds in cracks and crevices of walkways or patios.

- Use vinegar as a barrier to keep ants away from your patio or pool. You can also pour it around a sandbox to keep them away. Repeat after rain.

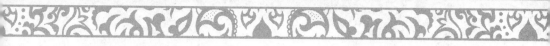

- Clean outdoor toys such as tricycles and sand toys using equal parts of water and vinegar. Sprinkle baking soda on badly soiled spots. Let it set for an hour and scrub. Rinse with water.

- Preserve cut flowers by adding two tablespoons of vinegar and one teaspoon of sugar to a quart of water.

- Keep cats out of your garden area by setting a sponge soaked in white vinegar in the dirt. As soon as the cat smells the vinegar, it will move on.

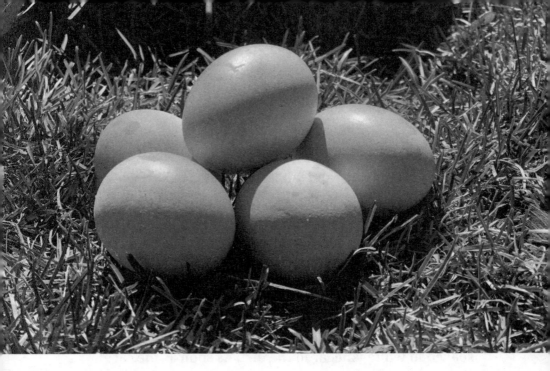

Fun Stuff

Chicken Leg Bender

Place a chicken leg or thigh bone in a glass of undiluted vinegar for about three days to make it bend like rubber.

Raw Egg Bouncer

Make a raw egg bounce by soaking it in a bowl of vinegar for two days. Rinse it off and astonish your friends.

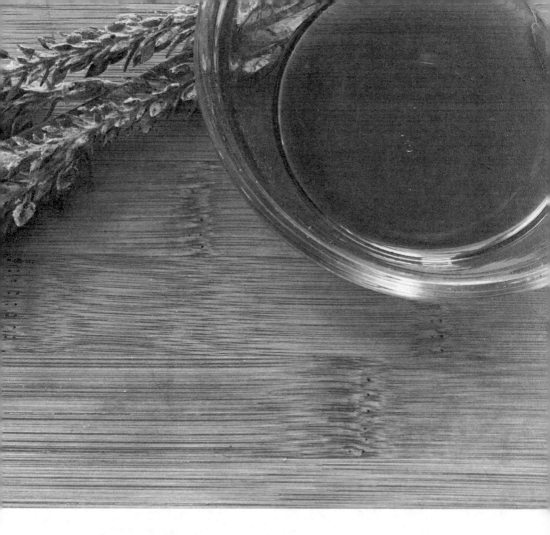

Crystal Garden

Grow this amazing garden with the help of vinegar.

1. Cut a sponge to fit inside the bottom of a shallow
    ceramic container.

2. Boil a cup of water and slowly add in 1/4 cup coarse
    salt. Stir while adding.

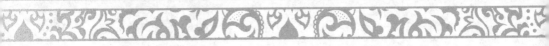

3.   Add two teaspoons of vinegar and stir well.

4.   Pour the mixture over the sponge so that there is a little liquid in the bottom of the container.

5.   Save the extra liquid and pour over when evaporation occurs.

6.   Watch closely and after a few days crystals will grow. Add food color to the solution if you want colorful crystals.

Penny Polisher

Polish pennies by soaking them overnight in a glass bowl full of vinegar. To speed up the process, boil the vinegar first.

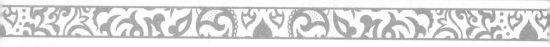

Easter Egg Dye

Make a lasting Easter egg dye by placing eggs in a solution of three cups boiling hot water, two tablespoons vinegar and food color of your choice. Re-dip eggs if needed to make the color bolder.

Vinegar Volcano

The young scientists in your home will love this project.

1. Fill an empty yogurt container 1/2 full with vinegar. Cut a 4-inch square piece of tissue paper and place one teaspoon of baking soda in it.

2. Pull the corners shut and twist the paper shut.

3. Drop it into the vinegar and watch!

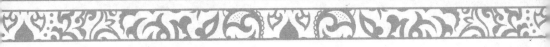

Wrapping Up

This guide has only scratched the surface when it comes to all the things you can do with vinegars. As old as time, vinegar offers countless possibilities for healing, beauty, food and more. If you are accustomed to making vinegars your sidekick in just the kitchen, it is time to spread your wings! Explore new and exciting types of vinegar and what they can do for you all around your home and garden.

Enjoy!